THE
POST-PREGNANCY
DIET

THE POST-PREGNANCY DIET

HOW TO REGAIN YOUR FIGURE AFTER YOUR BABY IS BORN

by
Susan Duff

With an Introduction by
Amy Glaser, M.D.

NAL BOOKS

NEW AMERICAN LIBRARY

A DIVISION OF PENGUIN BOOKS USA INC., NEW YORK
PUBLISHED IN CANADA BY
PENGUIN BOOKS CANADA LIMITED, MARKHAM, ONTARIO

NOTE TO THE READER

The ideas, procedures, and suggestions contained in this book are not intended as a substitute for consulting with your physician. All matters regarding your health require medical supervision.

Published simultaneously in Canada by
Penguin Books Canada Limited.

NAL TRADEMARK REG. U.S. PAT. OFF. AND FOREIGN COUNTRIES
REGISTERED TRADEMARK—MARCA REGISTRADA
HECHO EN DRESDEN, TN, U.S.A.

SIGNET, SIGNET CLASSIC, MENTOR, ONYX, PLUME, MERIDIAN and NAL BOOKS are published *in the United States* by New American Library, a division of Penguin Books USA Inc., 1633 Broadway, New York, New York 10019, *in Canada* by Penguin Books Canada Limited, 2801 John Street, Markham, Ontario L3R 1B4

Library of Congress Cataloging-in-Publication Data

Duff, Susan, 1945–
    The post-pregnancy diet : how to regain your figure after your baby is born / Susan Duff.
        p.   cm.
    ISBN 0-453-00595-0
    1. Reducing diets—Recipes. 2. Mothers—Nutrition. 3. Exercise for women. I. Title.
RM222.2.D727   1989
    613.2′5—dc19   88-8499
                                                                              CIP

First Printing, April, 1989

2   3   4   5   6   7   8   9

PRINTED IN THE UNITED STATES OF AMERICA

To Paul and Polly

Acknowledgments

I thank Dr. Amy Glaser for her important contributions to this book, as well as for her wisdom, energy, and friendship. For their enlightened expertise, I thank Charmaine Aleong and Marya Warshaw-Chu. For her initial support of this project, I thank Carole Hall, and for ongoing interest and inspiration, my editor at NAL, Alexia Dorszynski. For ideas, enthusiasm, and creative contributions, I'm grateful to my agent, Richard Pine, and I thank Dr. Leslie Blumberg, Barbara Cohen, Susan Eisner, Barbara Flanagan, Gay Haubner, Leah Ife, Martha Lorini, Shannon Miller, Sari Scheer, and Ellis Weiner. And, for keeping Polly entertained while I toiled, my heartfelt thanks to Celinda Andino, and to David Cohen, Lizzy Denis, Lauren Hamernick, Nick Ife, and Nat Weiner.

Contents

Introduction

Shortly after being asked to write an introduction to this book, I entered my office to give a prenatal class. Generally centered on infant feeding and newborn characteristics, this class has been helpful in allaying expectant couples' anxiety about the first two weeks at home with a new baby. On this particular evening, the first question came from a thirtyish man still three months from fatherhood: "How long before my wife returns to her [thin] pre-pregnancy figure?" There were knowing smiles all around the room. Clearly, he was not the only one concerned with this aspect of new parenthood.

Years ago, when I first came to the Park Slope section of Brooklyn to start a private practice, I enlisted a dancer acquaintance of mine to set up pre- and post-pregnancy exercise classes in the neighborhood—a concept I had thought quite innovative when I encountered it in my first practice. To my chagrin, I soon discovered there was no need. My friend already had three competitors in the area.

Although the pregnant couple may be very concerned about a woman's postpartum weight, there is minimal interest in it in the medical community, and little if any reference material in the medical literature. The relevant medical writings concentrate to a large extent on weight gain and nutrition during pregnancy and are perplexingly sparse in regard to weight loss postpartum.

During pregnancy, the fetus accounts for about ten to twelve pounds of the expectant mother's weight gain. Increased weight of uterine and breast tissue adds approximately five pounds, and the increase in blood volume another four pounds. The additional weight a woman gains is deposited as fat reserves to sustain fetal growth during the latter part of pregnancy, provide energy for labor and birth, and maintain lactation after birth. Most of the variation in weight gain among individuals reflects differences in expansion of maternal body fluids and fat stores.

As a medical patient, the overweight post-pregnant mother actually has no established practitioner to turn to. If there have been no complications in delivery, the obstetrician sees the mother again only at six weeks postpartum, primarily to assess her physical recovery from childbirth.

As a pediatrician, I may become involved in interpreting feelings of postpartum depression, or in support of breast-feeding, but generally, I am too concerned with weighing and measuring the newborn to notice the new mother's figure unless she mentions it herself. She rarely does.

I expect that the new mother of the eighties is somewhat reticent in asking for help with losing weight because she is so bent on being a super wife, mother, and career woman that she tends to view her weight gain as yet another aspect of her life that she is supposed to have complete control over.

What I have observed in my practice in a middle-class neighborhood of brownstones and co-ops is a very definite trend toward "super-motherhood." The mothers who bring their new babies to me for regular checkups are very much focused on doing everything perfectly for their infants. I know that these women are going through tremendous personal changes themselves, yet they rarely bring up issues concerning themselves.

If the postpartum woman herself is reluctant to mention so "petty" a complaint as an unexpected and unwanted weight gain, and the medical establishment seems to ignore the problem, the overweight new mother is left quite on her own to try to get back in shape. Given this woman's need to pursue a kind of perfection in everything she does at this stage in her life, her added pounds become a very pressing problem for her to solve alone. And, if she must return to her place of work, there is no question that she will be expected to look, as well as to perform, as she did before giving birth.

Who gains too much weight during pregnancy? Statistics reveal that younger women gain slightly more than older women; primiparous women (those giving birth for the first time) gain more than multigravidas (those delivering after a first birth); and thin women gain more than overweight women. Although these statistics offer a composite portrait of a younger, thinner woman, giving birth for the first time as the one finding herself with the post-pregnancy weight problem, my own practice reflects a different trend—that of the thirty-plus working woman giving birth for the first time. And, indeed, the latest data indicate postponement of childbearing to later ages, with first births to mothers between thirty and thirty-nine years of age being the most significant increase in birth rates in recent years. One must surmise that many if not most of these women have put off motherhood for career reasons, and that many if not most will return to careers after giving birth.

Pregnancy and motherhood represent a dramatic change in living habits for such a woman. Although previously she left the house before eight A.M. and returned at six or seven P.M., she now spends her early post-pregnancy weeks homebound and relatively more sedentary. She may be near her own kitchen twenty-four hours a day for the first time in her adult life, and she is likely to be sleeping and eating on an erratic schedule. She is apt to be fatigued as well. These combined circumstances make it quite difficult for a new mother to take off the extra weight she gained during pregnancy.

Endocrinologic—hormone—changes may also play a role in the difficulty of losing post-pregnancy weight. During pregnancy, progesterone regulates the deposit of fat, and it is possible that there is a delay in progesterone returning to the pre-pregnant level in the overweight postpartum woman.

One must remember that a woman brings to pregnancy all her previous experiences and conditions, and that, for a given individual, multiple factors of nutritional status, lifestyle, and hormones may all contribute to post-pregnancy weight problems.

A healthful and effective post-pregnancy diet seems long overdue, and I am pleased to see both recognition of the problem and intelligent solutions to it. In simplifying weight loss for the mother of the eighties and nineties who is busy trying to be perfect in every other sphere of her life, THE POST-PREGNANCY DIET addresses a crucial concern of many women who have given birth. It is my hope that this book will also serve as a reminder and an aid to medical clinicians as they deal with the very important personal needs of the post-pregnant woman.

—Amy Glaser, M.D.
Brooklyn, New York

Chapter 1

Gaining Too Much During Pregnancy and Trying to Lose It

When you become a mother, your life changes dramatically in lots of ways, and inevitably your body changes as well. For some women, the physical changes are minimal and short-lived. Within months or even weeks, they have miraculously returned to their pre-pregnancy shapes. Alas, for the rest of us, it's not quite as easy. All or some of the weight we gained during pregnancy stubbornly remains, clinging to our figures in unexpected places.

Pregnant women can gain anywhere from five to fifty (or more) pounds beyond the twenty-five to forty pounds health practitioners usually recommend that we gain during the nine-month term. Though some of the pregnancy weight may be lost when the baby is born, and some women report losing more quickly while breast-feeding, for many women the extra pregnancy pounds linger, sometimes for years. In my mother's day, the saying went that every child adds five (or was it ten?) pounds to a woman's figure. Most women today simply can't accept this as a fact of life.

Wanting to get back to "normal" as much as possible is a universal longing among all new mothers. There is an overwhelming desire to integrate the new and different person you have become—yourself as a new mother—into the life you lived before pregnancy. For most women, an important feature of that former life was their physical appearance—and principally, the shape of their bodies.

5

I know all about the problems involved in getting your figure back after your baby is born because I've experienced them myself. My experience is probably similar to yours in some ways. Here is my story:

I had dieted all my adult life until I became pregnant in my late thirties. On my first visit to the obstetrician, the doctor told me to stop dieting and to avoid gaining more than thirty pounds over the next nine months. I knew I couldn't do both.

In the past, my figure had ranged from slender to average to a few pounds over what I liked to weigh. But dieting had always been a way of life for me, and counting calories, combined with regular visits to exercise class, was the only way I knew to maintain the figure I liked to have. For me, "eating normally"—not dieting—meant certain weight gain.

Of course, I followed my doctor's orders and gave up dieting during my pregnancy. I also gave up smoking, and instead of my usual glass of wine with dinner, I often treated myself to a tasty dessert. By the time I was ready to give birth, I was forty pounds over my recommended pregnancy gain. Three months after the baby was born, I had forty pounds to lose.

I'd never before had to face losing more than a few pounds at a time. Now I was a new mom with more than just a few pounds to lose—and I needed lots of energy to care for the baby as well as to get back to work. I didn't have much time to devote to planning a nutritious, low-calorie diet and an effective exercise program. I needed an easy approach to weight loss that took into consideration a new mother's lifestyle. Most of all, I needed my pre-pregnancy figure back.

I searched in vain for a program to meet all the needs of a woman who had gained too much weight during pregnancy and wanted to lose the extra pounds as soon as possible after giving birth. To my surprise, I found only a few post-pregnancy exercise books. And like most women who have had experience with trying to lose weight, I knew I couldn't lose my fifty post-pregnancy pounds with exercise alone.

It was then that I decided to summon all the knowledge of weight loss I'd garnered during my fifteen-year career as a syndicated diet columnist and writer to create my own program for taking off the weight that lingers after pregnancy. I knew it would be a difficult task given my situation—my new and different health needs as a new mother and the extreme time constraints now imposed on my daily life by the added responsibilities and compelling pleasures of being a parent. I wanted to share what I learned with all the other women in my situation. This book is the result.

First, I tackled my own weight problem from a nutritional angle. I consulted with nutritionist Charmaine Aleong, a registered nurse with a degree in nutrition, to find out how I could get all the nutrients a new mother needs and at the same time keep calories low enough to lose excess pounds.

From the beginning, Charmaine emphasized that it's *essential* for new mothers to be well nourished from the moment they give birth. She told me that although individual cases may vary, many nutritionists estimate that, after giving birth, the body requires *eighteen months* to regain the healthy nutritional status that is depleted during pregnancy. Because good nutrition is so important to a woman's sense of mental and physical well-being, the diet of a new mother is definitely related to her stress levels and her ability to cope. "Diets that emphasize quick weight loss may be tempting for the overweight new mother," Charmaine told me, "but a lack of nutritional balance is especially unsafe during the post-pregnancy period. Temporary weight loss may be achieved, but it will leave you feeling tired, irritable, and less able to deal with all the new stresses in your life. This is dangerous for your own health and may interfere with your ability to care for your child properly." Charmaine also reminded me that most diets won't correct the poor eating habits that may have contributed to extra weight gain during pregnancy, and many women gain back lost weight when eating behavior has not been changed.

It became clear to us that we needed to devise a diet that offered excellent nutrition, sure and steady weight reduction, and a re-education in eating behavior. Our diet had to be designed to become part of a permanent healthy lifestyle suitable for all women who gained too much during pregnancy, no matter when their babies were born. I also wanted to add a feature to our diet: a program to help women get control of their appetites again. Many of us are enormously hungry during the nine months of pregnancy, or during some part of that period. After the delivery, that hunger often tends to linger; like a habit that's hard to break.

We solved this problem by adding a period of abstinence from sugar to the front end of the diet. Before you begin the formal diet meal plans, you must abstain from all sugar for three days—including the "hidden" sugar contained in many popular prepared foods and condiments. I think you'll be amazed at the way this one simple sacrifice helps cut down your appetite and prepares you for the continuing changes in your eating behavior involved in the formal diet plan.

Charmaine and I started working on this diet when my daughter was three months old. Our overall approach to reducing calories and providing plenty of good nourishment for my new mother's body was to cut back on the high-calorie refined sugars and fats. At one point, we minimized the diet's fat content so severely that the eating plan became *too* fat-free. From years of reporting on diets, I had thought that the less fat one consumed, the better, but Charmaine reminded me that the right amount of fatty acids is a wholesome and necessary feature of any healthy diet. We solved the problem by adding one tablespoon of corn oil or corn oil margarine to each day's menu.

I have always preferred the kind of diets that don't require exact measuring and weighing of foods; being so exacting with portions seems to me to add to the kitchen-work tedium of dieting, and it didn't seem fair to add yet another tiresome chore to a new mother's already busy schedule. Unfortunately, some nutritious and essential elements of a healthy diet are simply too high in calories to be taken in unlimited portions. We had to limit the amounts of certain protein and complex carbohydrate foods (meat, poultry, and even fish, plus pasta, rice, and bread) in order to keep the diet's calories low. Almost all the vegetables on the diet, however, can be enjoyed in unlimited amounts during mealtimes.

Charmaine and I agreed that the best structure for a weight-reduction diet for new mothers was one based on three meals a day. The traditional schedule of breakfast, lunch, and dinner seems to fit in best with a mother's daily pace and helps establish a regular eating pattern for the whole family. Also, because I had become accustomed to snacking throughout the day during my pregnancy, I needed to break the habit and readjust my appetite to a schedule of three squares a day. I thought other new mothers as well could benefit from the behavior modification involved in limiting eating to three well-spaced times of day, and no between-meal snacks, with one exception.

Because we wanted to add extra calcium to the diet, and because we wanted to make the diet easier for new mothers who may have gotten used to eating more often during pregnancy, Charmaine and I ultimately added one between-meals snack to the diet, a delicious high-calcium drink we call the New Mom's Milkshake. This very satisfying shake seemed a good way of helping wean new mothers from their pregnancy habit of snacking, while adding a good calcium boost to the diet at a very low calorie count.

This drink proved a truly successful addition to the diet. It's not really a snack, because it's a liquid, and yet it's so good-tasting and filling that it really helps you make it through a hungry period between meals. You may enjoy it at any time of day—mid-morning, mid-afternoon, or before bed. I think you'll find as I did that it helps you feel a little more pampered and a little less deprived while you're dieting.

Working full-time at my career and having a young child doesn't leave me much time for creative meal preparation, but like many women, I enjoy cooking when I can experiment with different combinations of seasonings and other ingredients. I didn't want this diet to demand lots of time in the kitchen on the part of new mothers, because that usually means time away from our families in the evening. On the other hand, I didn't want to ask dieters to follow exacting recipes for every meal, no matter how efficient the recipes might be.

To make the diet more flexible and to make food preparation appealing both to the experimental cook and to the woman who is more comfortable reading a recipe, I have designed the meal plans so that you can either prepare the foods as you would like (using the Permitted Ingredients Lists as a guide to what you can add) or follow the recipes offered with the diet meal plans. You can also elaborate on the given recipes by adding anything you like from the Permitted Ingredients Lists, or by subtracting ingredients you don't care for. I think you'll find that this diet suits a variety of individual cooking styles. And, you can enjoy preparing your diet meals in either way without having to spend much time in the kitchen.

As the diet began to take shape, Charmaine and I felt satisfied that we were meeting the specific criteria for a good-nutrition, low-calorie new mother's diet. Meals call for everyday foods that even nondieting husbands will enjoy; and, because all meal plans are listed for you and all nutritional and caloric calculations are done for you,

you have one less thing to think about—that is, *what to have for dinner*, or even for breakfast or lunch.

By the time Charmaine and I had worked out all the details of the diet and felt it was just about perfect, my daughter was nine months old. The diet was ready to be tried, and I was more than ready to start trying to get my pre-pregnancy figure back. But, there was one problem: I was still breast-feeding.

Almost every expert opinion we came across at this point discouraged us from even attempting to tackle the problem of making our diet appropriate for nursing mothers. It seemed that there were too many individual variables among women who breast-feed, and that caloric needs varied widely from one nursing mother to another.

The standard guidelines are that lactating women require an extra five hundred to six hundred calories per day to produce sufficient milk for an infant whose sole source of nourishment is mother's milk. But, some women may require more calories to keep their milk supply up, while others will need fewer calories—and the caloric requirements will vary even more according to different babies' feeding patterns and the addition of supplemental sources of nourishment for the infant.

I felt very strongly about developing a diet that would work for breast-feeding mothers without jeopardizing their milk supply. I was still nursing my baby at nine months and I had no immediate plans to stop. I knew that half of all the women in America breast-feed during some part of their children's infancy, and I was sure that among them there were many women who, like me, were anxious to start trying to take off extra pregnancy weight.

I became terribly discouraged at this point in my work on this project. I really wanted to start getting my figure back, but I was afraid that a diet that provided only about a thousand calories a day might adversely affect my milk supply. Also, I honestly doubted my own willpower. The baby was eating some solid foods and she wasn't nursing as frequently as she had six months ago, but I felt ravenous during the whole period I was breast-feeding. I was afraid that even a nutritious and satisfying diet such as the one Charmaine and I had designed would be difficult for me while my hunger level was so high.

I decided I'd just have to wait until I weaned the baby before I could start dieting seriously, and I resolved to be patient in the meantime. It was a difficult period for me. I loved breast-feeding and I didn't want to cut it any shorter than I had to, but I was growing increasingly uncomfortable with all the extra pounds I was still carrying around. I knew there must be lots of other women who were feeling just as I did at that point in motherhood.

It wasn't until five months later, when my daughter was fourteen months old and I had just weaned her that Charmaine and I finally hit on a solution—an ingenious one that allows each breast-feeding mother who wants to lose weight to work out her own individual diet plan, by adding special treats that raise calcium and protein intake to the levels necessary for a nursing mom, and allow her to adjust her calorie intake to her individual needs.

We call these additions to the diet Supplemental Snacks for Breast-feeding Moms. Each nursing mother should follow the Post-Pregnancy Diet as it is written, adding to the meal plans two New Mom's Milkshakes a day, and one or two of the ten snacks listed. You'll need to show this plan to your doctor or health care practitioner so you can work out the right combination of shakes and snacks to add to your diet at the beginning, but you'll be able to adjust your caloric intake to suit your own needs by adding or subtracting the supplemental snacks.

I think this system will work beautifully for breast-feeding mothers. It allows you lots of extra food when you are hungriest, adds extra protein and calcium to your daily nutrient intake, and lets you gradually reduce the number of snacks as you wean your baby. Best of all, it means you can lose weight slowly and healthfully, while you're breast-feeding, without interfering with the quality or quantity of your baby's milk supply.

The Post-Pregnancy Diet with Supplemental Snacks for Breast-feeding Moms will probably give you more nutrient value than what you are eating now, *and* it will help you gradually begin losing weight as soon as you want to start. But do show Chapter 3, "Guidelines for Nursing Mothers," to your medical professional to get her approval before you begin, and ask for specific recommendations.

My baby was about fifteen months old, and completely weaned, by the time I started the diet. For the first two months, I followed the Post-Pregnancy Diet in earnest and I felt wonderful, full of energy and stamina. I won't say I was never hungry, but I was so inspired by how steadily I was losing weight that my willpower was at an all-time high. Two or three weeks into the diet, I knew my eating behavior was undergoing a major change—my between-meals hunger diminished enormously, sweets and fatty foods no longer appealed to me, and in general, I thought about food much less than I ever had before. There was no need to think much about food since all my meals were already planned for me, and all I had to do was glance at my diet chart to know what I was to eat for breakfast, lunch, and dinner.

There was one aspect of the diet that I particularly liked, although it had not been intentionally planned: Now that my daughter was a toddler and often ate at the table with my husband and me, she often asked for (or grabbed) the foods we were eating. For the most part, we could share what was on our plates—our Post-Pregnancy Diet meals—with her.

The original diet plan that I was following then included lots of special reduced-calorie or "diet" foods—mayonnaise, salad dressing, diet soda, diet margarine. These foods often had too many chemical additives in them for me to feel comfortable giving them to Polly. I had always thought these diet products were a great way to keep calories down and still eat more or less normally. Before I became pregnant, I used to spend a good deal of time in the grocery store checking labels to find the lowest calorie counts. (During my pregnancy, of course, I checked labels to try to find foods that didn't contain chemicals or coloring agents, so I had to reject all my favorite diet foods.) Like many women, I had relied on these products to help me cut calories in my earlier dieting days, and once I'd had the baby and was ready to start dieting again, I was ready to rely on them again. But it seemed unfair, as well as inconvenient, to be eating things at the table that I couldn't share with Polly.

All this gave rise to what must be a very frequent revelation for many new mothers: My zealous concern for the healthy, wholesome quality of the food I was giving to my small daughter made me think twice about what I was eating myself. I had been careful to eat nothing but natural fresh foods when I was pregnant (only the very best pastries and chocolates would do for me in those days!), and I was as careful about feeding Polly nothing but the healthiest foods now, but I was much less cautious about what I was willing to feed myself. Suddenly, it just didn't seem to make sense to be using diet products again.

At that point, after two months of dieting, I had lost about fourteen pounds following the Post-Pregnancy Diet, as it was written then, with lots of diet foods included. I certainly wasn't ready to stop dieting, or to stop losing, but I knew that Charmaine and I had to revamp our diet yet again to find alternatives to the diet foods I'd originally insisted on having.

My final approach to the problem was to combine some old diet know-how with some new experiments in the kitchen. Low-fat cottage cheese is delicious spread on whole wheat toast in the morning and provides more calcium than diet margarine. Lemon juice or vinegar sprinkled on fresh or cooked vegetables seems to bring out their natural good taste much more than the artificial flavorings in most diet dressings. When I felt that a hot vegetable required something just a little bit gooey to dress it up, I found a tablespoon of grated parmesan cheese really did the trick—and it added extra calcium to the meal. For a creamy pasta mixer, I came to love low-fat yogurt or cottage cheese, both of which increase calcium and have low calorie counts.

I quickly became accustomed to this new style of eating, and I soon really liked the way foods tasted: fresher, cleaner, more natural and wholesome. It was also great to feel free to let Polly have whatever she wanted from among the foods I was eating at mealtimes.

On my first week of the new Post-Pregnancy Diet, I lost three pounds, almost twice as much as I had been losing per week on our previous version of the diet. Charmaine thought this might have been because so many of the diet foods are high in sodium, which can cause water retention. I hardly cared about the reasons; I was enjoying the diet more than ever, and losing more efficiently than before.

Seventeen pounds slimmer, buying pretty new clothes for the first time since my pregnancy, I was feeling more confident than ever in the Post-Pregnancy Diet. So confident, in fact, that I wanted to add two new features to the diet that seemed slightly daring. First, I wanted to add a glass of wine to the evening meal. And second, I wanted to be able to go off the diet on weekends so I could socialize more freely.

Although Charmaine always approached our diet from an academic nutritionist's point of view, she was also very open to my ideas about making the diet less drastic, more humane, and more compatible with the everyday life of a mother with young children. I thought we new moms needed something special at the end of the day, and a glass of wine with dinner seemed the perfect little treat to look forward to.

I confess that I'm a great fan of wine, and an evening meal without it made me feel deprived. Our diet already included a piece of fresh fruit as desert after dinner; couldn't we let new moms substitute a glass of wine with dinner for the fruit desert when they wished to, I wondered. Charmaine went over the diet carefully and decided that, yes, wine could be substituted for fruit at the evening meal without seriously affecting the high nutritional value of the diet.

Over the next week, I experimented with adding the lovely indulgence of wine with dinner to the diet, and I found it made a wonderful difference. One evening, when Polly had eaten and gone to bed early, my husband and I had a peaceful meal alone together, and the glass of wine allowed me to linger at the table without having my thoughts drift to longings for a rich dessert. Another time, when we had dinner with Polly, my glass of wine made our little gathering a bit more civilized than it might otherwise have been (with our child pouring her juice on the floor and flinging broccoli hither and yon). Two evenings just didn't lend themselves to wine with dinner, and on those occasions, I was delighted to collapse in the living room after supper with a piece of fresh fruit to munch while I watched the TV news and my husband read Polly to sleep.

At the end of that experimental week, with four "with wine" dinners and three fruit-for-dessert dinners, I'd lost one and a half pounds. I knew that wine had a few more calories than fruit (the average for a glass of wine is about one hundred calories, for a piece of fruit, about seventy-five), but there were evenings when the wine really meant a lot to me, and I was willing to increase my calorie intake a little in order to enjoy this evening indulgence. I realize, of course, that not everyone likes wine as much as I do, and that some dieters will opt for fruit on a regular basis. Those of you who enjoy a nice glass of wine with dinner will find this a very welcome and different feature of the Post-Pregnancy Diet, however.

Wine has also been included in some of the diet recipes, and on the Permitted Ingredients List, for those who like to cook with wine. (Cooking burns off all the alcohol and most of the calories in wine, so it can be used quite liberally in diet cooking.) Those who prefer not to use wine at all will find there are other liquids they can substitute in the recipes calling for wine.

My glass of wine is one thing I can't share with Polly at our evening meals, of course, but she quickly accepted this when I let her sniff my glass a few times to demonstrate that she wouldn't really like it. "Mommy's wine, no-no" was one of the first clearly spoken phrases, and naturally, it always came up at the most inappropriate times.

Nursing mothers should consult with their pediatricians on the advisability of a glass of wine with dinner. Many doctors seem to feel that a nursing mother's occasional glass of wine with dinner is not in any way harmful to her breastfeeding child, but check with your own doctor to be sure. (My own experience was that my glass of red wine with dinner sometimes seemed to irritate Polly's stomach a bit the next morning so I gave it up until she was weaned.)

Having a mini-vacation from your formal diet on the weekends was an idea that also appealed to me tremendously. No matter how good-tasting and satisfying and convenient a program of diet meals may be, Saturdays and Sundays are the days when most of us want to break away from routine, enjoy some unstructured time, meet friends for meals. All these weekend pleasures seem even more important when you have a child and the workaday week is, by necessity, a series of rigidly scheduled days.

Yet, as everyone who's ever dieted has probably learned, going off your diet on the weekend often means regaining all those pounds you lost during your diet week.

Charmaine and I started talking about how we could work out a system whereby dieters could go off the formal diet on weekends without re-gaining lost weight.

First we considered establishing a return to the sugar abstinence period every weekend. But we knew that even without any sugar at all on Saturday and Sunday, there would still be serious pitfalls for the dieter, most of them falling into the category of fats. It was then that we realized that if we allowed dieters to take a break from the formal diet plan with only two restrictions on their eating—no sugar, no extra fats—we could enable them to have quite a bit of freedom, without promoting weight gain over the two-day period.

Charmaine found this idea very attractive. She felt it could be an exercise in behavior modification for dieters: They could test the new eating habits they were learning during the five-day formal diet period and discover for themselves how they could modify their everyday eating simply by following two simple rules—without the structure of set meal plans on the weekends. She also felt confident that with this system most dieters would either continue losing or, at worst, maintain their weight. It seemed an ideal solution.

Over the next month, I experimented with the new, new, Post-Pregnancy Diet as a five-day formal meal plan diet followed by two days of eating as I liked—but without sugar or added fats. On my first weekend off with guidelines, I lost a half a pound; the second weekend, I maintained my weight; the third weekend, I lost one pound, and the fourth weekend, I maintained again. By the end of the month, I'd lost six and a half pounds, and I was thrilled with the way our weekends-off system was working.

I found that I prepared many of my favorite Post-Pregnancy Diet meals when we ate at home over the weekend, just because it was easiest to follow a set meal plan, but I'd switch around the vegetables, or have dinner at noon on a Sunday, or have only the New Mom's Milk-shake for lunch on a busy Saturday. Invitations to a friend's home for dinner or brunch sometimes presented problems, but I found ways to solve them (see Weekend Strategies, p. 82). After five days of following diet meal plans exactly, I was definitely in a "dieting mode," and having some freedom on the weekends made the diet much easier to stick with, without the anxiety of re-gaining weight.

Knowing that most women who work outside their homes eat out during the week for at least a few of their meals, I'd already made provisions in the diet for eating in restaurants. Our restaurant lunch and dinner selection lists, already part of the diet, worked beautifully for week-end socializing in restaurants as well.

At this point, Charmaine and I felt we had designed a wonderful diet for new mothers: Nutrient values were very high, to help women regain the depleted nutritional status that follows pregnancy; calories were low to pro-mote steady and efficient weight loss; our program in-cluded good behavior modification techniques to help dieters retrain their eating habits; and we'd included lots of features to make this the kind of diet that was very compatible with a post-pregnancy lifestyle.

Best of all, I'd lost a total of twenty-five pounds, and I finally felt that I was getting back to normal, getting my pre-pregnancy figure back, that the end was in sight, just fifteen pounds more to lose.

I kept thinking about the one element of our weight-loss program I'd been neglecting: exercise. From the be-ginning, Charmaine had emphasized how important it was to include regular physical activity in our weight-loss program. I knew from writing about dieting and from reading about weight loss that when you cut back on calories for a period of time, your metabolism eventually adjusts to the new calorie count and you stop losing weight. I also knew that exercise was essential to continual, permanent weight loss because it steps up the pace of your metabolism so you can use calories more efficiently. And I was very aware that regular aerobic exercise had other benefits important to weight loss, that it helped reduce your appetite to make dieting easier, and that it toned and firmed your body as the pounds came off.

Despite knowing all this I kept putting off my search for a good exercise program for new mothers. I simply couldn't imagine how I, or any new mother, could possibly find the extra time in a day to devote to exercise. Working full time at my career and spending every spare second with my daughter and my husband, I used whatever extra and rare moments I found to myself to collapse in exhaustion, glance at a newspaper, return a friend's phone call. I had no idea how new mothers could manage to muster the energy or allocate the required number of hours per week to get enough exercise. And, besides, I was still losing quite well on my diet.

Then, in the midst of resisting the inevitable, my diet hit a plateau. Though I continued to follow the diet to the letter, I went for five days without losing a pound. Over the next two days, without so much as a thought to something that wasn't on the diet, I gained a pound. What I had known to be true theoretically was in fact proving itself true within my body. Perhaps because I had started the diet at a weight so much greater than my normal body weight, I had managed to lose twenty-five pounds in a three-and-a-half-month period, but I now knew I couldn't continue to lose with diet alone. My metabolism had adjusted to the lowered calorie count, and I would have to begin a good program of regular exercise to take off the last fifteen pounds.

My search for the perfect exercise consultant for my post-pregnancy weight-reduction program soon led to Marya Warshaw-Chu. In my residential family neighborhood, Marya was famous for her pre- and postnatal exercise classes in a beautiful, light-filled studio.

My first visit to one of Marya's postnatal classes was a sheer act of courage. I had not really exercised since the midpoint in my pregnancy, over two years before. Since I was a "beginner," I was in a class with women who had given birth as recently as a few months earlier. Many brought their infants with them to class, which added a pleasant and unintimidating atmosphere.

One of the great advantages of going out to a postnatal exercise class is that it puts you in touch with mothers like yourself who feel their bodies have changed as a result of pregnancy and who want to get back in shape. I had believed that my weight gain and overall out-of-condition status were unusual in the midst of our cultural fascination with diet and fitness. It was reassuring and comforting to meet other women who had also overgained and let themselves get out of shape during pregnancy and new motherhood.

After trying out a few of Marya's postnatal classes, I signed up for her "Spring Intensive" series, with classes given at various times every day of the week. I knew that forcing myself to get moving every day could really shake up my metabolism, and I hoped it would start me losing again. I was right. Even at my advanced stage of dieting, when it's often hardest to lose the last pounds, I took off two and a half pounds the first week and two pounds the second. Even better, I was beginning to feel parts of my body that I hadn't really been in touch with for a long time.

In just two weeks, my post-pregnancy jelly-belly started to firm up. My buttocks and thighs felt leaner, more toned. I began to regain the flexibility in my spine that allows more everyday ease in movement. My posture improved, and that made my figure look better right away. I wanted other new and not-so-new-but-out-of-shape mothers to experience the same wonderful benefits of Marya's class, so I was delighted when she agreed to participate in the Post-Pregnancy Diet and Exercise Program. Chapter 6, "The Stages-of-Motherhood Guide to Exercise," takes you through Marya's complete postnatal class for students four weeks or more postpartum. There are even some of Marya's special exercises that some women will be able to start within weeks of delivery (with their doctor's or midwife's permission, of course), and some especially rigorous exercises to add to your routine once your baby is six months old. And, if you think you don't have time to exercise at all, Marya's special ten-minutes-a-day approach is guaranteed to put you on the road to movement, no matter how busy you are.

Getting started on an exercise program that really made my body feel better helped me regain tone and firmness where I needed it, *and* gave my diet the boost it needed to become the real beginning of a more physical lifestyle. Once I became involved in a program of physical activity, I couldn't imagine *not* making time for exercise, no matter how overfull my days seemed. Also, I had known all along that I would need to add some aerobics to my personal exercise program.

Almost all diet experts agree that some form of aerobic activity as a regular and consistent element of lifestyle is essential to the ongoing success of a weight-loss diet program. This undeniable fact continues to be demonstrated in new findings on the subject. While Marya's postnatal exercise program offers many benefits in toning, firming, strengthening, and enhancing flexibility, it is not an aerobic routine, since it doesn't raise the output level of the heart and lungs for a sustained period of time. You will need to supplement this routine with an aerobic activity of your choice.

There are many appealing aerobic exercises to choose from. Ideally, you will want an activity that keeps you moving for a sustained half-hour to forty-five-minute period, one that you can do regularly, at least three times a week. For most new mothers, the choice of an activity will involve different elements of a lifestyle relating to your and your child's schedule. See Chapter 6 for suggestions.

In my case, with a child starting nursery school, a stationary bike proved the most convenient and enduring aerobic activity. (I tried taking a half-hour jog after walking Polly to school some mornings, but that tended to upset my mornings and set my workday back too much— by the time I'd showered and gotten to my desk, there was too little time left for me to accomplish anything before picking Polly up at school for lunch.) My ultimate solution to fitting an aerobic routine into my life was to set up the stationary bike in our bedroom. I'd get Polly up in the morning, set her up in my bed with breakfast on a tray, and pedal away on my bike for forty-five minutes while we both watched *Sesame Street* and chatted about the day. More often than not, I took Polly to school wearing the crummy old sweats I'd been biking in, but on a few very well-organized mornings, I could manage to shower and dress before walking her to school. In any case, biking in the morning was a routine I could stick with at least three or four days a week, and it seemed to work for me.

My own experience with aerobics and diet proved all the truths that are already known: Aerobic exercise helps you lose weight faster and more continually, helps cut your appetite, adds to your stamina and energy, and is really worth the extra time you have to set aside for it.

When I was about finished writing this book, I realized that I was still a few pounds above my pre-pregnancy weight, that I hadn't quite arrived at my original goal. I remembered that several doctors I'd consulted with on the subject of post-pregnancy weight suggested that I might never achieve the figure I had before I got pregnant. Just as our lives change when children are born into a family, our bodies may also be changed in some small but permanent way.

For many new mothers, achievement of the ideal goal

will be relatively quick and easy. Others may find that at some point they have to accept an extra few pounds, or an extra few inches, or an extra bit of softness here and there. The diet-and-exercise program in this book will help you get as close as is physically possible to your pre-pregnancy body, and most of you will probably end up with exactly the figure you had before you became pregnant. But all new mothers should be prepared to accept the ways their bodies may have changed. The whole philosophy of this book is to help you learn how to work *with* your new post-pregnancy body. It's important that you feel respectful and caring toward your body no matter *what* shape you're in when you begin this program.

I know this is a weight-loss system that works, one that will help every new mother get her figure back. I hope you find it an easy and enjoyable program to follow. I think you will, and I wish you all the very best of luck!

Chapter 2

The Diet

About the Diet

New mothers have a different set of diet problems, and that's why we need a special diet that's tailor-made for all the ways our bodies and our lives have changed. This diet has been specially formulated by a nutritionist to meet the nutritional needs of a woman who has given birth—and to help her lose the extra pounds gained during pregnancy at the same time. In addition, it is a diet designed to help very busy new moms simplify food preparation and mealtimes.

As you can see from looking over the Post-Pregnancy Diet ten-day meal plan (with weekends off!) on the following pages, nutritional and caloric calculations have all been done for you. Your daily calorie counts amount to about 1,000 to 1,200 calories a day, and all the nourishment a mother who has recently given birth needs is packed into the delicious diet meals you are offered.

If you are breast-feeding, you needn't put off dieting until you have weaned your baby. Special guidelines and supplements at the end of the chapter show you how you can stick to this diet by adding some delicious snacks while continuing to breast-feed your child.

You'll find the Post-Pregnancy Diet easy to integrate into normal family mealtimes, and you won't have to make separate dishes for your husband or the new baby's

25

older siblings. All the diet meals here include normal wholesome dishes that everyone can enjoy.

The five-day diet meal plans specify amounts for one portion, and most vegetables can be eaten in unlimited amounts. To include your husband and other family members, simply multiply the single-portion quantities. (The recipe section offers recipes that serve two and may be doubled, or added to.)

You can formally begin the Post-Pregnancy Diet by following the sugar abstinence program (as outlined later) for three days, beginning on a Friday. (Make it *this Friday*.) Over the course of the weekend take time to look over the meal plans. Make a shopping list of the foods and ingredients you will need for the next five days. Do your marketing a day or two before the Monday you plan to begin dieting so you will have everything you need on hand. On the third day of sugar abstinence, the day before you begin the diet, look over the meal plans again, and start planning how you'll prepare your meals.

Plan ahead in other ways as well. For the first two weeks of dieting, avoid eating out in restaurants or at a friend's home; you'll want to follow the diet exactly during this beginning period. After the first two weeks of dieting, you may eat out as often as you want, by referring to the alternate restaurant lunches and dinners you can substitute for that day's diet meal. You can eat out at friends' homes by following the weekend guidelines. But get used to this healthful new way of eating by sticking to the diet exactly as it's written for the first two weeks.

This diet is structured to provide you with all the nutrients you need at this stage in your life, with lowered calorie counts to help you lose weight. It simplifies your eating so much that it practically does the dieting for you. At the same time, there is enough flexibility built in so that you can have a normal social life of eating out while you're dieting.

Start sugar abstinence this Friday, then begin your diet the following Monday. You're on your way at last to your pre-pregnancy figure!

About Sugar Abstinence

One of the most difficult problems encountered by those of us who want to diet after having a baby is that our appetites seem much larger than they've ever been before. During pregnancy, many of us ate more than usual, and developed new eating habits. Perhaps we got used to greater quantities of food, or maybe we ate more frequently. These habits are difficult to shake after the baby arrives. Even though you're only eating for one again, you may have retained some of that pregnancy eating behavior. And now those extra calories aren't going to your growing unborn child, but rather to the maintenance of your own extra body fat.

To combat this very common post-pregnancy eating syndrome, this diet helps to wean you from pregnancy eating behavior. The key is a three-day period of sugar abstinence. It's very simple to follow. For the three days prior to starting the Post-Pregnancy Diet, you will eat as you normally do, with one important exception: You may not eat any sugar; you may not add sugar to foods or eat foods containing sugar.

Three-day sugar abstinence helps new mothers in two ways. First, in most cases, it helps to reduce your overall appetite. By the end of a three-day period of not eating any sugar, you will almost certainly discover that you are significantly less hungry. This is a special bonus to those of us who have been pregnant, because it helps adjust our appetites to our current lowered calorie needs.

Second, abstaining from sugar for three days helps in

another important way: It teaches you to start controlling your eating behavior. For many of us who gained too much weight during pregnancy, out-of-control eating habits have become entrenched in our daily routines. Three-day sugar abstinence offers dieters a simple task that enables us to control one aspect of eating behavior—the elimination of all sugar—and this serves as an important training period before starting the diet.

Even if you don't think you eat much sugar, focusing on this one element of your diet will serve to prepare you for the diet to come. Also, you're apt to discover that there's more sugar in many of your favorite foods than you think. Once you start checking labels on processed foods, you'll find sugars cropping up in foods you don't normally think of as sweet—crackers and some bread, catsup, prepared sauces, relishes, pickles, juices, peanut butter. When you're checking labels, look for ingredients such as sucrose, molasses, dextrose, lactose, fructose and corn sweeteners—all are considered sugars.

Your three days without sugar will show you that you are able to monitor and change the way you eat, and this will enable you to start your diet with high self-confidence and strong motivation. By the end of the three-day period, you will find that your appetite has been decreased; you will have proven to yourself that you *can* control your eating, and you will be highly motivated to begin the more challenging task of sticking to a formalized diet meal plan.

Best of all, three-day sugar abstinence helps new mothers overcome one of dieting's most difficult obstacles: procrastination. There's no reason why you can't begin abstaining from sugar almost immediately—the very next Friday on your calendar, as a matter of fact. And, that will give you three days to get ready to start your Post-Pregnancy Diet on the following Monday. It couldn't be easier!

Getting Started

Eat as you normally do, with two exceptions: Do not add to food or beverages any refined or raw white or brown sugar, or honey, and do not eat any foods or beverages containing any sugar, refined or raw, white or brown, or any honey. Check labels of all processed foods to look for hidden sugar ingredients, which may be listed as sucrose, molasses, lactose, fructose, or corn sweeteners; all of these are sugars and the foods containing them should be avoided during sugar abstinence. If you do not have access to the package of a food and cannot check the ingredients listing, *do not eat it* unless you are absolutely sure it contains no sugar. Begin sugar abstinence on Friday; the following Monday, begin the Post-Pregnancy Diet, your first step toward getting back to your pre-motherhood figure.

Many new mothers will lose weight during the sugar abstinence period; some will not. Keep in mind that the point of this introductory phase of the Post-Pregnancy Diet is to start conditioning your appetite and modifying your eating behavior so that the diet itself will be easier for you. If you do start to lose weight during your three-day sugar abstinence, consider it yet another bonus of this super-easy, very effective eating plan for new moms.

The Post-Pregnancy Diet

Two Five-Day Menu Plans
for Two Weeks of Easy Dieting

Follow this diet exactly as written for the next five days. In addition to the foods listed for each day's meal plan, have one New Mom's Milkshake as a snack every day (see recipe for milkshake, p. 43). After five days on the diet, take the weekend off, following the special guidelines. For the next five days, follow the diet exactly as written, then take the weekend off, again following the special guidelines. The next day, begin the diet plan again with Day 1 meal plans.

If you have questions about the diet or if you want more information about food preparation, see the sections following the five-day menu plans: "Permitted Ingredients for Dinner Preparation," "Definition of Food Terms," "Permitted Fruits List," "Post-Pregnancy Diet Rules," and "The Post-Pregnancy Diet Dinner Menus with Recipes."

If you will be having lunch and/or dinner away from home, refer to "Take-Along Lunches," "Restaurant Lunches," and "Restaurant Dinners."

If you are breast-feeding, refer to Chapter 3, "Guidelines for Nursing Mothers."

Week 1 ⌒

Day 1

BREAKFAST   ½ grapefruit
or
¼ cantaloupe
or
¼ honeydew
or
1 orange, quartered
1 thin slice whole wheat or protein toast
¼ cup low-fat cottage cheese, sprinkled with
     cinnamon
plain tea or coffee

LUNCH   Sandwich ingredients:
2 thin slices low-fat or part-skim cheese
     (1 ounce)
sliced tomato
1 tablespoon mustard
lettuce leaves
1 whole wheat pita bread pocket
6–8 oz. tomato or vegetable juice

DINNER   6 oz. boneless chicken breast, poached in
     chicken broth
1 small baked potato with 1 tablespoon
     corn oil margarine and chives
steamed broccoli with lemon wedges
1 4-oz. glass of wine
or
1 piece of fruit

Day 2

BREAKFAST   1 large biscuit shredded wheat
or
1 cup mini shredded wheat
½ cup skim milk
1 medium peach, sliced, or ½ banana, sliced,
    or ½ cup berries
plain tea or coffee

LUNCH   Combine:
1 cup cooked (⅔ cup uncooked) whole wheat
    or spinach pasta
½ cup low-fat cottage cheese
1 small tomato, chopped
fresh or dried dill weed
dash pepper
mineral water, seltzer, or tea

DINNER   6 oz. lamb chop, broiled
1 steamed artichoke* with 1 tablespoon
    melted corn oil margarine and lemon
    wedges (for dipping)
steamed cauliflower with 1 tablespoon
    parmesan cheese
1 4-oz. glass of wine
or
1 piece of fruit

---

*If artichokes are not available, substitute brussels sprouts or asparagus, as much as you like.

Day 3

BREAKFAST   ½ grapefruit
or
¼ cantaloupe
or
¼ honeydew
or
1 orange, quartered
1 thin slice whole wheat or protein toast
¼ cup low-fat cottage cheese, sprinkled with
    cinnamon
plain tea or coffee

LUNCH   Combine:
1 3½-oz. can or half a 7½-oz. can pink or
    red salmon
1 stick celery, finely chopped
1 tablespoon lemon juice and 1 teaspoon
    mustard, whisked together
1 whole wheat pita bread pocket
1 slice (1 oz.) part-skim, low-fat mozzarella
    cheese
(Put cheese into pita bread; heat at 300°F.
    for 5 minutes; fill pita pocket with salmon
    mixture.)

6–8 oz. tomato or vegetable juice

DINNER   4–5 oz. lean chopped beef mixed with
    minced onion
sliced green pepper
steamed sliced carrots with 1 tablespoon
    corn oil margarine and sprinkling of
    cinnamon
1 4-oz. glass of wine
or
1 piece of fruit

Day 4

BREAKFAST   1 large biscuit shredded wheat
or
1 cup mini shredded wheat
½ cup skim milk
1 medium peach, sliced, or ½ banana, sliced,
    or ½ cup berries
plain tea or coffee

LUNCH   Combine:
lettuce and chopped parsley
sliced green pepper
1 small tomato
1 slice (1 oz.) low-fat, part-skim mozza-
    rella, cut in narrow strips
raw mushrooms, sliced
scallion or onion slices
½ cup lemon juice and 1 teaspoon mustard
    whisked together and poured over salad
mineral water, seltzer, or tea

DINNER   6 oz. veal chop, broiled
steamed spinach with 1 tablespoon corn oil
    margarine
⅔ cup cooked brown or white rice (¼ cup
    uncooked) with fresh parsley
1 4-oz. glass of wine
or
1 piece of fruit

Day 5

BREAKFAST   ½ grapefruit
or
¼ cantaloupe
or
¼ honeydew
or
1 orange, quartered
1 thin slice whole wheat toast
¼ cup low-fat cottage cheese, sprinkled with
    cinnamon
plain tea or coffee

LUNCH   1 cup chicken noodle soup
1 thin slice whole wheat bread, topped with
    ½ small tomato, sliced, and
1 slice (1 oz.) part-skim mozzarella cheese
mineral water, seltzer or tea
Note: You may broil the bread, tomato,
and cheese for 3 minutes.

DINNER   6 oz. baked or broiled fish or shellfish with
    lemon juice and herbs
lettuce and tomato with wine vinegar, salt,
    and pepper
green beans with 1 tablespoon corn oil
    margarine
1 4-oz. glass of wine
or
1 piece of fruit

Days 6 and 7

TAKE THE WEEKEND OFF!

Follow these simple guidelines:

1. No refined or raw sugar or honey, or foods containing refined or raw sugar or honey.

2. No fats or foods containing fats or oil. Trim all visible fat from meats, remove skin from poultry. No cream, no butter or cheese, no dairy foods. No added fats or oils when cooking, except one tablespoon corn oil margarine or corn oil daily. See Chapter 4, "Weekend Strategies and Forbidden Foods."

3. No snacking; no between-meals nibbling. Eat three separate meals a day, plus your New Mom's Milkshake. If you are nursing, you may choose from among the supplement snacks to add to your three daily meals and New Mom's Milkshakes.

Week 2 ⌇

Day 1

BREAKFAST   1 large biscuit shredded wheat
or
1 cup mini shredded wheat
½ cup skim milk
1 medium peach, sliced, or ½ banana, sliced,
    or ½ cup berries
plain tea or coffee

LUNCH   Sandwich ingredients:
3½ oz. water-packed tuna
lettuce leaves
mustard
one whole wheat pita bread pocket
6–8 oz. tomato or vegetable juice

DINNER   6 oz. lean London broil
1 baked potato with low-fat yogurt and
    chives
lettuce, cucumber, fresh coriander and/or
    parsley, topped with lemon juice
whisked with 1 tablespoon corn oil
1 4-oz. glass of wine
or
1 piece of fruit

Day 2

BREAKFAST   ½ grapefruit
or
¼ cantaloupe
or
¼ honeydew
or
1 orange, quartered
1 thin slice whole wheat toast
¼ cup low-fat cottage cheese
plain tea or coffee

LUNCH   Sandwich ingredients:
1 oz. low-fat cheese
tomato slices
lettuce leaves
cucumber slices
one whole wheat pita bread pocket
mineral water, seltzer or tea

DINNER   6 oz. baked or broiled fish or shellfish
sliced tomatoes
steamed, chopped broccoli, chilled and
    tossed in salad with lettuce, onion slices,
    1 tablespoon corn oil, and freshly squeezed
    lemon juice, plus herbs of choice
1 4-oz. glass of wine
or
1 piece of fruit

Day 3

BREAKFAST   1 large biscuit shredded wheat
or
1 cup shredded mini-wheat
½ cup skim milk
1 medium peach, sliced, or ½ banana, sliced,
    or ½ cup berries
plain tea or coffee

LUNCH   Combine:
1 cup cooked (⅔ cup uncooked) whole wheat
    or spinach pasta
½ cup low-fat yogurt
chopped cucumber and tomato
mineral water, seltzer, or tea

DINNER   ½ chicken breast, baked or broiled (remove
    skin before cooking)
lettuce, onion, parsley, with 1 tablespoon
    corn oil and wine vinegar
green beans with 1 tablespoon grated
    parmesan
1 4-oz. glass of wine
or
1 piece of fruit

Day 4

BREAKFAST
½ grapefruit
or
¼ cantaloupe
or
¼ honeydew
or
1 orange, quartered
1 thin slice whole wheat toast
¼ cup low-fat cottage cheese, sprinkled with cinnamon
plain tea or coffee

LUNCH
Open-face sandwich ingredients:
1 slice (2 oz.) lean ham
1 slice (1 oz.) low-fat, part-skim mozzarella cheese
tomato slices
mustard
1 slice whole wheat or protein toast
mineral water, seltzer, or tea

Note: You may broil the prepared sandwich for 3 minutes.

DINNER
6 oz. turkey breast or lean ground turkey
salad of raw greens and tomato, with 1 tablespoon corn oil and vinegar
½ cup cooked (⅓ cup uncooked) whole wheat or spinach pasta, with 1 tablespoon grated parmesan
1 4-oz. glass of wine
or
1 piece of fruit

Day 5

BREAKFAST
1 large biscuit shredded wheat
or
1 cup mini shredded wheat
½ cup skim milk
1 medium peach, sliced, or ½ banana, sliced,
   or ½ cup berries
plain tea or coffee

LUNCH
Salade niçoise ingredients:
3½ oz. water-packed tuna
lettuce and parsley
sliced cucumber
wine vinegar and mustard, whisked together
mineral water, seltzer, or tea

DINNER
6 oz. fish or shellfish, baked or broiled,
   with lemon juice and herbs
⅔ cup (¼ cup uncooked) steamed brown or
   white rice with fresh parsley
lettuce, carrot curls, sliced radishes, with 1
   tablespoon corn oil and wine vinegar
1 4-oz. glass of wine
or
1 piece of fruit

Days 6 and 7

TAKE THE WEEKEND OFF!

Follow these guidelines:

1. No refined or raw sugar or honey, or foods containing refined or raw sugar or honey.

2. No fats or foods containing fats or oil. Trim all visible fat from meats, remove skin from poultry. No cream, no butter or cheese. No added fats or oils when cooking, except one tablespoon corn oil margarine or corn oil daily. See Chapter 4, "Weekend Strategies and Forbidden Foods."

3. No snacking; no between-meals nibbling. Eat three separate meals a day, plus your New Mom's Milkshake. If you are nursing, you may choose from among the supplement snacks to add to your three daily meals and New Mom's Milkshakes.

After the weekend, you may start again with the Post-Pregnancy Diet meal plan for Week 1, Day 1, and continue dieting until you have arrived at your weight goal.

Everyday Snack

New Mom's Milkshake

6 ice cubes
½ cup cold water
5 tablespoons nonfat dry milk powder
½ teaspoon vanilla
dash cinnamon
***fruit, cut into 1-inch pieces**

Blend all ingredients at high speed for 45 seconds to one minute. Be sure your blender can safely handle ice cubes. Pour into a 10-oz. glass. Enjoy.

*FRUIT OPTIONS:
  ½ banana
  1 small apple, or pear, or peach (cored or pitted, peeled or with skin)
  ½ cup berries
  ¼ cantaloupe or honeydew, skin and seeds removed
  1 tangerine, or ½ orange, peeled and seeded

Choose only one fruit option for each daily milkshake.

If you would like to add additional fiber to your diet, you may add one tablespoon Miller's bran to blender before blending milkshake.

Permitted Ingredients
for Dinner Preparation

Unlimited Ingredients

You may use as much of these ingredients as you like when preparing your meals, and you may add any of the permitted raw vegetables to your plate at mealtime. But you may add these ingredients *only* at dinner; you are not permitted to snack on them between meals.

Liquids

Vinegar: Wine, cider, white, or flavored with herbs
Mustard: Yellow, brown, Dijon, coarse, or flavored with herbs, onions, or wine
Lemon or lime juice: Fresh or bottled (unsweetened)
Chicken or beef broth or consommé: Canned, home-made (all fat skimmed), reconstituted from cubes or granules
Nonstick spray coatings (such as PAM)
Tomato juice, or mixed vegetable juice (such as V-8)

Seasonings

Pepper: Red, white, or black; coarse or fine
Cinnamon
All green herbs, fresh or dried
Curry powder or cumin
Nutmeg: Excellent sprinkled on top of New Mom's Milkshake
Hot pepper flakes, hot pepper sauce

Fresh Raw Vegetables

Celery
Carrots
Green pepper
Radishes
Mushrooms
Garlic
Onion
Scallions
Shallots
Leeks
Chives
Bean sprouts

Limited Ingredients for Dinner Preparation

You may add the amounts specified here *for each portion* of a dinner dish.

¼ cup dry wine, white or red
¼ cup low-fat plain yogurt
1 tablespoon soy sauce
1 tablespoon grated parmesan cheese
½ cup skim milk

Definition of Food Terms

Wine: Must be dry, unfortified, unsweetened table wine, no sherry, wine coolers, or port.

Bread: Pita or any whole-grain, thin-sliced, diet protein bread; no more than eighty calories per slice (check calorie count on label).

Pasta: Any macaroni, spaghetti, fettucine, or other pasta, fresh, frozen, or dried, in any shape or size. Spinach, carrot, and whole wheat pasta offer extra nutrients at no extra calories. *No egg noodles; no filled pasta,* such as ravioli, tortellini, stuffed shells; *no frozen pasta* prepared with sauce or cheese; *no boxed macaroni-and-cheese mixes.* These pastas are all higher in calories than the standard.

Vegetables: May be fresh or frozen, without sauce; served raw, steamed, boiled, or baked without added fats (unless corn oil margarine is specified).

Low-fat cottage cheese: Carton should state that the product is low-fat; look for the percentage of milkfat, which should be 2 percent or less.

Low-fat yogurt: Carton should state that the product is plain, low-fat yogurt (no sugared or fruit-flavored yogurt is permitted); look for the percentage of milkfat, which should be 1.5 percent milkfat or less.

Permitted Fruits List

Following are the amounts of fruits that constitute one portion, which you may have following your evening meal when you choose not to have wine. All fruits must be fresh—neither canned nor frozen with syrup.

½ banana
1 small apple, or pear, or peach
1 cup berries (blueberries, raspberries, strawberries, blackberries)
½ cup green or red grapes
¼ cantaloupe or honeydew melon
1 orange, tangerine, or tangelo
2 plums
1 kiwi

2 apricots
½ cup cherries
½ papaya
½ mango
¼ pineapple

Post-Pregnancy Diet Rules

• Wherever quantities or weights of foods or ingredients are specified, you must measure or weigh each portion; where no quantities or weights are specified, you may prepare and enjoy as much as you like of the food or add as much as you like of the ingredient. Note: Pasta and rice should be measured *after cooking*; weigh meat, chicken, and fish *before cooking*.

• Have one New Mom's Milkshake every day; nursing mothers, see "Guidelines for Nursing Mothers" at chapter's end. You may have your milkshake at any time of day—mid-morning, mid-afternoon, before bed.

• Where exact fruit portions are not specified, as in "one piece of fruit," in dinner menus, you may have one serving of any of the permitted fruits: one apple, one peach, one pear, one nectarine, half a banana, one tangerine, one orange, two plums, one kiwi, one cup of strawberries, blueberries, grapes, blackberries, raspberries, or a quarter of a cantaloupe or honeydew melon.

• Begin the diet on a Monday; eat all the meal plans as specified, plus one New Mom's Milkshake every day.

• Have your nightly glass of wine *with* your dinner, rather than before the meal. (Studies show that wine before a meal tends to increase the appetite, while wine with a meal helps you eat less.)

• Try to plan your schedule so that there are three to four hours between meals. Eat all the foods specified at one sitting, during the meal. Do not save portions of a meal to eat between meals.

• Drink water, club soda, or seltzer with lemon or lime wedges throughout the day, as much as you like. Try to have four to six eight-ounce glasses each day in addition to what is specified on the diet.

• For the first two weeks of dieting, try everything specified on the diet, even if you think you won't like it. When you are permitted unlimited quantities of foods, eat until you are satisfied; you needn't scrimp on the unlimited portions of vegetables listed in lunch and dinner menus. Eat as much as your hunger dictates, but stop as soon as you are full.

• Prepare foods as you wish, using ingredients from the Permitted Ingredients List (you may add as much of these ingredients as you like), or try the recipes for dinner menus in the recipe section that follows. These recipes may be altered or varied to suit your taste, as long as you use ingredients on the Permitted Ingredients List.

• Each meal offers a grouping of foods; you may combine these foods if you wish—at breakfast, for example, you may scoop cottage cheese onto a melon wedge, or spread whole wheat toast with cottage cheese. At lunch, you may fill pita bread with other foods to make a sandwich, or you can enjoy the foods individually for your meal. Some combinations are obvious. Most people will prefer to add milk and fruit to cereal; salads are more enjoyable when vegetables are tossed together. When pasta is listed as a lunchtime meal, it is best combined with the other foods listed, such as yogurt, vegetables, etc.

- Follow the diet exactly as specified for the first two weeks —the two five-day diets, and weekends off with guidelines. This will be easiest for you if you are still at home with your baby—a good motivation to start the diet now! If you have begun working outside your home, see the section on take-along lunches, and for the next two weeks, make plans not to eat out in restaurants. If you often have business lunches, try to reschedule them for early-evening "drinks dates" when you can order only seltzer or club soda. After you have followed the diet exactly as it is written for two weeks, you may eat out in restaurants; see the section on restaurant lunches and dinners, and substitute these meals for the meals listed on the diet as necessary.

- After the first two weeks on the diet, you may also eat out at a friend's home, on a Saturday or Sunday, while strictly adhering to the weekend guidelines—no sugar, no fats.

- Take any vitamin and/or mineral tablets or supplements recommended by your physician. In addition, it is recommended that you take 500 milligrams of calcium lactate daily. (Recent research confirms that we require 1,200 milligrams of calcium per day to prevent osteoporosis; the Post-Pregnancy Diet is high in dietary calcium but no healthful diet has sufficient levels to meet this high daily requirement.)

- Weigh yourself every day if you like; you'll lose fast on this diet, and weighing-in provides a tangible reward for your dieting efforts. Best time to weigh: as soon as you wake up, before eating or drinking anything.

The Post-Pregnancy Diet
Dinner Menus with Recipes

The five-day menu plans on the preceding pages outlined for you the foods you can enjoy three meals a day on this diet. Breakfast and lunch foods can be prepared and eaten as you like them, either by combining the foods listed or having them individually. The Permitted Ingredients lists following the menu plans allow you to create your own slimming dinner recipes and dishes by preparing in your own way the foods listed for the evening meal on any given day. Especially as you begin this diet, however, you might prefer to follow exact recipes when you make your first diet dinners.

The Post-Pregnancy Diet recipes are designed to show you a new way of preparing dinner with favorite everyday foods combined in delicious ways to minimize both fat and calories. Even if you really love to do your own creative cooking, try the recipes that follow at least once. Using the Permitted Ingredients lists, you can add or substitute your own personal choice of ingredients, as you choose. These recipes can stimulate your culinary creativity by offering you new ideas in diet cooking.

All in all, this diet is designed to offer you as much variety as possible while you're dieting. There are lots of different recipes here, and you'll learn many new ways to enjoy preparing food in this healthful way. It's also the intention of this diet to offer you flexibility. If you're really rushed one night, you might find it easier to follow the dinner recipe given here for that particular diet day. In a more leisurely mood when your baby or child goes to bed early, you might want to try some more creative cooking, using the recipes as a starting point. When you switch back and forth between following the meal plans and using the recipes, just be sure to stick to the meal

plan or menu given for that specific diet day; it's important that you follow the sequence of the meals on this
diet from one day to the next.

Here are some pointers for using the recipes:

- All the recipes here are for two adult servings. They
  may be halved, doubled, or tripled to suit your family size. The vegetable portions on this diet are unlimited; in the following recipes, specific amounts are
  given as guidelines. These amounts may be adjusted
  to suit your and your family's appetites. For toddlers
  and preschoolers, two-ounce portions of meat, chicken,
  or fish are suggested, and two- to three-ounce portions of vegetables, rice, and pasta.

- You may use spices to taste. In most cases, the mea-
  sures for spices in these recipes are for medium- to
  well-spiced food. None of the recipes includes salt.
  You may add salt to taste at the table, but to reduce
  water retention while you diet, it's best to keep salt
  to a minimum and avoid using it in cooking altogether.

- Recipes for cooked vegetables always specify steam-
  ing rather than boiling. This is because vegetables
  lose some nutrients when they are in contact with
  water during cooking, and you'll want to get all the
  nourishment value of all the food you eat on **this**
  diet. A collapsible steamer basket is a small invest-
  ment, and invaluable to diet cooking.

- When part-skim mozzarella cheese is specified in a
  recipe, you may substitute any part-skim or low-fat
  cheese you like. When parmesan cheese is specified,
  you may substitute another hard, grated cheese, such
  as romano.

- Some of the recipes for preparing dinner include wine
  as an ingredient. Wine is an excellent flavoring agent
  in cooking, and since the alcohol burns off during

cooking, it adds taste without adding significant calories. If you'd like to use the suggested recipes but you'd prefer not to include wine, you may substitute an equal amount of water or broth (vegetable, chicken, beef) to provide adequate liquid for cooking.

• If you will be using the recipes, or variations of them, regularly, look over the five-day dinner menus at the beginning of each week to make sure you have on hand all the staples, such as seasonings and vegetables, that may not be included on the five-day meal plans. The dinner menus with recipes are basically the same as the meal plans, but may occasionally call for extra ingredients. Plan ahead so you'll have everything you need at the ready.

Recipes

Week 1 ◡‿つ
Day 1 Dinner Menu

Wine Poached Chicken
Baked Potato with Chives
Lemon-Cayenne Broccoli
Dry red or white table wine (4-ounce glass)
or
¼ cantaloupe

Wine Poached Chicken
(serves 2)

1 cup chicken broth (homemade, canned, or from bouillon
  cube or granules)
2 cups water
½ cup dry white table wine
1 large carrot, pared and cut crosswise into four pieces
1 medium onion, peeled, and quartered
½ teaspoon freshly ground pepper
1 tablespoon dried parsley
1 12-ounce chicken breast, split, boned, skin and fat removed

Place broth, water, wine, carrot, onion, pepper, and parsley in a large, heavy saucepan. Bring to a boil over high
heat. Place two chicken breast halves into boiling pot;
reduce heat and simmer chicken for 15 minutes. Remove
immediately; serve with cooked vegetables from the pot.

Baked Potato with Chives

2 baking potatoes
2 tablespoons corn oil margarine
2 tablespoons fresh chopped chives

Preheat oven to 400° F. Scrub potatoes and prick each
twice with a fork. Place in oven to bake for 45 minutes.
Slit open skin and place 1 tablespoon corn oil margarine
in each hot potato. Sprinkle 1 tablespoon chives over
each open potato.

Lemon-Cayenne Broccoli

4 large stalks fresh broccoli
½ teaspoon grated lemon rind
Juice of one lemon
¼ teaspoon ground red pepper, or cayenne

Trim and rinse broccoli. Place in steamer basket over boiling water, cover, and steam for ten minutes. In small bowl, stir together grated lemon rind, lemon juice, and cayenne. Pour mixture over cooked broccoli.

Day 2 Dinner Menu

Savory Lamb Chops
Artichokes with "Lemon Butter"
Parmesan Cauliflower
Dry red or white table wine (4-ounce glass)
or
1 peach

Savory Lamb Chops
(serves 2)

2 6-ounce lamb chops, any cut, bone in, all visible fat removed
2 large cloves garlic
1 tablespoon dried rosemary

Peel garlic cloves and cut each in half lengthwise. Season both chops as follows: Rub cut side of garlic over one side of lamb chop; turn chop and rub the other side with the other half of garlic clove. Take a pinch of rosemary and distribute over both sides of each chop, crumbling the leaves between your fingers as you sprinkle.

Preheat oven broiler for 5 minutes. Place chop on raised broiling rack; broil 6 to 8 minutes per side for rare to medium one- to one-and-a-half-inch thick chop.

Artichokes with "Lemon Butter"

2 large artichokes*
2 tablespoons corn oil margarine
Juice of one lemon

Trim stem and leaf tips from artichokes, then place them in steamer basket over boiling water, cover, and steam for 30 minutes. Melt margarine in small saucepan. Add lemon juice, and stir to combine. Pour "lemon butter" into a small bowl to serve as a dipping sauce for artichokes.

Parmesan Cauliflower

½ cauliflower head, cut into bite-sized pieces
2 tablespoons grated parmesan cheese

Rinse cauliflower pieces and place them in steamer basket over boiling water; cover and steam for 15 minutes. Toss hot cauliflower with grated cheese and serve.

*If artichokes are unavailable, you may substitute brussels sprouts or asparagus; drizzle "lemon butter" over hot, cooked vegetable.

Day 3 Dinner Menu

Stuffed Peppers Italiano
Cinnamon Carrots
Dry red or white table wine (4-ounce glass)
or
1 apple

Stuffed Peppers Italiano
(serves 2)

1 large green pepper
Nonstick spray coating
½ pound very lean chopped beef
1 small onion, peeled and coarsely chopped
1 tablespoon dried oregano
1 tablespoon dried basil
⅛ teaspoon freshly ground black pepper
1 cup tomato or V-8 juice
2 tablespoons shredded or grated part-skim mozzarella cheese

Cut green pepper in half lengthwise; remove stem, seeds, and white membranes; rinse halves well. Place pepper halves in steamer basket over boiling water; cover and steam for 5 minutes. Spray heavy, 10-inch skillet with nonstick spray coating; add to skillet chopped beef, onion, and seasonings; brown over low heat for 15 minutes, stirring occasionally. Pour tomato juice over meat mixture; stir and cook over low heat 5 minutes more. Place cooked pepper halves in shallow baking pan; spoon meat mixture into peppers, dividing evenly between two halves. Top each meat-filled pepper half with 1 tablespoon mozzarella. Bake in preheated 350°F. oven for 10 minutes.

Cinnamon Carrots

4 to 5 medium-sized carrots
2 tablespoons corn oil margarine
½ teaspoon cinnamon

Wash and pare carrots; remove tops and slice into ¼-inch disks. Place carrot slices in steamer basket over boiling water, cover, and steam for 8 to 10 minutes. Toss hot carrot slices with margarine and cinnamon, stirring to evenly distribute; serve immediately.

Day 4 Dinner Menu

Dijon Veal Chops
Rice with Parsley
Spinach au Gratin
Dry red or white table wine (4-ounce glass)
or
1 fresh orange

Dijon Veal Chops
(serves 2)

½ cup chicken broth (homemade, or canned, from bouillon cube or granules)
½ cup white wine
1 teaspoon Dijon or yellow mustard
1 stalk scallion, white part only, sliced very thin (reserve green stem)
2 veal chops, 6 to 8 ounces each, with bone in, all visible fat removed
6 to 8 medium-size fresh mushrooms

Preheat oven to 350° F. In large measuring cup combine broth, white wine, and mustard; stir briskly with a fork to combine. Add sliced scallion. Place veal chops in a shallow baking pan. Trim, rinse, and slice mushrooms; distribute evenly over veal chops. Pour mustard sauce over chops and mushrooms. Bake in preheated 350° F. oven for 30 minutes. Serve immediately over rice; spoon mushrooms and sauce over chops.

Rice with Parsley

2 ⅔-cup servings of rice (instant, white, or brown) prepared according to package directions
1 scallion, green stalk only
1 teaspoon dried parsley

Thinly slice the scallion stalk; add with dried parsley to hot, cooked rice, and toss to mix in greens.

Spinach au Gratin

6 cups fresh spinach, or one 10-ounce package frozen spinach, chopped or whole leaf
2 tablespoons corn oil margarine
2 tablespoons grated parmesan cheese

Rinse and cut stems from fresh spinach, place in steamer basket over boiling water; cover, and steam for 5 to 8 minutes; or, prepare frozen spinach according to package directions. Toss hot spinach with margarine, sprinkle with cheese, cover, and keep warm until served.

Day 5 Dinner Menu

Lemon-Garlic Grilled Fish Steaks
Garden Salad
Green Beans Parmesan
Dry red or white table wine (4-ounce glass)
or
1 nectarine

Lemon-Garlic Grilled Fish Steaks
(serves 2)

2 6-ounce salmon or swordfish steaks
2 lemons
1 small clove garlic
2 tablespoons fresh minced parsley
⅛ teaspoon freshly ground black pepper

Grate lemon rind to make 1 teaspoon grated lemon rind.
Squeeze juice from both lemons; remove seeds. Combine
rind and juice in large measuring cup. Press garlic clove
into juice mixture; add parsley and black pepper; stir with
a fork to combine. Heat oven broiler for 5 minutes. Place
fish steaks on broiler pan; pour half of lemon sauce over
steaks. Broil fish 6 inches from heat source 3 to 4 minutes;
turn. Pour remaining sauce over fish; broil 3 to 4 minutes.

Garden Salad

1 small head green leafy lettuce
2 medium tomatoes
6 fresh mushrooms
4 scallion stalks
juice of one lemon
¼ cup basalmic or wine vinegar
½ teaspoon dry mustard
⅛ teaspoon freshly ground black pepper

Rinse lettuce well and tear into bite-sized pieces; place in medium-size salad bowl. Wash and stem tomatoes; cut into quarters, then halve the quarters. Wash, trim, and slice mushrooms. Trim ends of scallions and slice white and green parts. Combine lemon juice with vinegar; stir in dry mustard and pepper. Toss vegetables together in salad bowl; add lemon-vinegar dressing, toss again.

Italian Green Beans

3 cups fresh string beans
2 tablespoons corn oil margarine
2 tablespoons grated parmesan cheese
1 tablespoon dried oregano

Wash and trim beans. Place them in steamer basket over boiling water; cover, and steam for 10 minutes. Toss hot cooked beans with margarine, cheese, and oregano; serve hot.

Week 2 ⌒
Day 1 Dinner Menu

Barbecued Steak
Baked Potato with Chive Dressing
Crispy Green Salad
Dry red or white table wine (4-ounce glass)
or
2 plums

Barbecued Steak

(serves 2)

This recipe calls for preplanning and requires 2 hours marinating time.

12-ounce London broil, all visible fat trimmed
1 cup tomato or V-8 juice
2 tablespoons wine vinegar
1 tablespoon prepared spicy mustard
1 tablespoon soy sauce
1 large clove garlic
½ teaspoon freshly ground black pepper

Combine tomato juice, vinegar, mustard, and soy sauce in a small bowl; press garlic clove into mixture; add pepper. Stir to mix well. Place meat in a shallow dish; pour sauce over, and marinate in the refrigerator for at least two hours (may be marinated overnight), turning the meat over once. Preheat oven broiler for 10 minutes. Broil meat on raised rack 6 inches from heat source for 7 to 10 minutes on a side.

Baked Potato with Chive Dressing

2 baking potatoes
½ cup plain low-fat yogurt
1 tablespoon freeze-dried chives

Preheat oven to 400° F. Scrub potatoes and prick each twice with a fork. Place in oven; bake 45 minutes. In small bowl, combine yogurt and chives. Slit open skin of hot, baked potatoes and spoon in chive dressing.

Crispy Green Salad

1 small head green leafy lettuce
1 large cucumber
¼ cup fresh coriander or parsley
2 tablespoons corn oil
¾ cup fresh lemon juice

Rinse lettuce well, and tear into bite-sized pieces; place in salad bowl. Pare and trim ends of cucumber; halve lengthwise, then cut into slices. Coarsely chop coriander or parsley. Place cucumber and greens in salad bowl. Briskly stir together corn oil and lemon juice. Toss vegetables and herbs together in salad bowl; add dressing and toss again.

Day 2 Dinner Menu

Paper-Wrapped Fish Fillet
Herb-Baked Tomatoes
Curried Broccoli
Dry red or white table wine (4-ounce glass)
or
¼ honeydew melon

Paper-Wrapped Fish Fillets
(serves 2)

2 6-ounce fish fillets, such as sole or bass, about ½-inch thick
1 small stalk celery
2 thin slices onion
4 tablespoons white wine

Preheat oven to 350° F. Rinse celery; trim ends and remove leaves; cut stalk in half crosswise, then cut narrow strips lengthwise. Tear off 2 10-inch lengths from 12-inch-wide roll of aluminum foil. Place one fish fillet in the center of each foil rectangle. Distribute celery strips evenly over fillets; place onion slice over celery. Top each vegetable-covered fillet with 2 tablespoons wine. Fold edges of foil together to form center seam across fillet; fold top and bottom edges of foil together to seal ends. Place foil-wrapped fish on oven rack and bake at 350° F. in preheated oven for 8 to 12 minutes. Open foil to serve.

Herb-Baked Tomatoes

4 medium tomatoes
non-stick spray coating
1 tablespoon fresh minced parsley (or 1 teaspoon dried parsley)
1 tablespoon fresh minced basil (or 1 teaspoon dried basil)
⅛ teaspoon freshly ground black pepper
2 tablespoons grated parmesan

Preheat oven to 350° F. Rinse tomatoes and remove stems; cut each tomato into 3 thick slices. Spray shallow baking dish with non-stick spray coating and place tomato slices in dish. Sprinkle herbs, pepper, and cheese on slices. Bake for 10 minutes.

Curried Broccoli

4 large spears broccoli
2 tablespoons corn oil margarine
½ teaspoon mild curry powder

Rinse and trim broccoli; place spears in steamer basket over boiling water; cover, and steam for 15 minutes. Melt margarine in small saucepan; stir in curry powder. Drizzle over cooked broccoli.

Day 3 Dinner Menu

Lemon-Mustard Chicken Breast
Tangy Salad
Green Beans with Cheese
Dry red or white table wine (4-ounce glass)
or
1 tangerine

Lemon-Mustard Chicken Breast

(serves 2)

2 small (6-ounce) chicken breasts
or
1 large (12-ounce) breast, split
1 cup chicken broth (homemade, canned, or from bouillon
    cube or granules)
juice of 1 lemon
1 teaspoon Dijon or tangy yellow mustard

Preheat oven to 350° F. Remove all skin and fat from chicken breasts; place in shallow baking dish. Combine chicken broth, lemon juice, and mustard in a large measuring cup; stir briskly with a fork. Pour lemon-mustard sauce over chicken breasts, and bake for 45 minutes.

Tangy Salad

1 small head leafy lettuce
1 small red onion
¼ cup fresh parsley
2 tablespoons corn oil
¼ cup tarragon-flavored wine vinegar

Rinse lettuce and tear leaves into bite-size pieces. Slice onion into very thin slices; separate rings. Coarsely chop parsley. Toss lettuce pieces, onion rings, and parsley together. Combine oil with vinegar; whisk or stir briskly with a fork. Pour dressing over salad; toss again.

Green Beans with Cheese

3 cups string beans
2 tablespoons grated or shredded part-skim mozzarella, or other low-fat cheese

Rinse and trim beans; place in steamer basket over boiling water; cover, and steam for 10 minutes. Toss hot, cooked beans with cheese and serve immediately.

Day 4 Dinner Menu

Grilled Turkey Patties
Primavera Salad
Cheese and Herb Pasta
Dry red or white table wine (4-ounce glass)
or
1 kiwi fruit

Grilled Turkey Patties
(serves 2)

12 ounces ground turkey
2 stalks celery
1 small green pepper
1 small onion
1 tablespoon soy sauce
⅛ teaspoon ground black pepper

Trim and rinse celery, green pepper, and onion; chop very fine. Place vegetables in large bowl with ground turkey; add soy sauce and ground black pepper. Mix ingredients, using hands to combine turkey and vegetables well. Form two large patties. Preheat oven broiler for 5 minutes. Place turkey patties on raised rack; broil 10 minutes on each side.

Primavera Salad

1 small head green leafy lettuce
2 medium tomatoes
2 medium carrots
2 scallions
2 tablespoons corn oil
2 tablespoons tarragon-flavored wine vinegar
2 tablespoons lemon juice
½ teaspoon Dijon or tangy yellow mustard
⅛ teaspoon freshly ground black pepper

Rinse lettuce and tear into bite-size pieces; place in salad bowl. Wash and stem tomatoes; cut into quarters, then halve the quarters. Rinse and pare carrots; remove tops, then use parer to cut into carrot curls. Thinly slice white and green parts of scallion. Toss tomatoes, carrots, and scallion with lettuce in salad bowl. Combine corn oil, vinegar, and lemon juice with mustard and pepper; stir briskly with a fork or whisk. Pour over vegetables and toss again.

Cheese and Herb Pasta

⅔ cup uncooked spinach or whole wheat pasta (any shape)
2 teaspoon fresh parsley, chopped fine
½ teaspoon dried oregano
½ teaspoon dried basil
2 tablespoons grated parmesan cheese

Cook pasta according to package directions. Drain and toss while hot with parsley, oregano, basil, and cheese until herbs and cheese are well distributed. Serve hot.

Day 5 Dinner Menu

Shrimp and Mushroom Toss
Curried Rice
Sunshine Salad
Dry red or white table wine (4-ounce glass)
or
½ grapefruit

Shrimp and Mushroom Toss
(serves 2)

½ **pound medium-size shrimp**
½ **pound medium-size fresh mushrooms**
juice of 2 lemons
2 teaspoons fresh parsley, chopped fine
⅛ **teaspoon freshly ground black pepper**

Rinse shrimp in cold water and place in steamer basket over boiling water; cover and steam for 7 minutes. Rinse again under cold water; remove shells and devein. Wash, trim, and slice mushrooms. Place in medium-size bowl with prepared shrimp. Pour lemon juice over shrimp and mushrooms; add parsley and black pepper. Toss together, and serve, or chill, covered, for half an hour.

Curried Rice

2 ⅔-cup servings of rice (white, instant, or brown), prepared according to package directions
1 scallion
½ **teaspoon mild curry powder**

Slice thinly green and white parts of scallion. Stir into hot cooked rice with curry powder; serve immediately.

Sunshine Salad

1 small head green leafy lettuce
10 radishes
1 medium cucumber
2 tablespoons corn oil
1 tablespoon grated lemon rind
Juice of one lemon

Rinse lettuce and tear into bite-size pieces; place in salad bowl. Rinse well, trim, and thinly slice radishes. Trim and pare cucumber; cut in half lengthwise, and slice thin. Toss radish and cucumber with lettuce pieces in bowl. Combine corn oil, lemon rind, and lemon juice, stirring briskly with a whisk or fork. Pour dressing over vegetables; toss together.

Take-Along Lunches

For those new mothers who can't be home for lunch but can brown-bag their noontime meals, the Post-Pregnancy Diet provides alternative take-along lunches. You can take them to your place of work, or to play group gatherings, or have picnics outdoors with your children.

There are five take-along lunches here. If you will be brown-bagging it to work every day, follow the sequence of the lunches as specified, from Day 1 through Day 5. If you will only be taking your lunch along on an occasional basis, it is best to prepare and take the lunch corresponding to the day of the week; Day 1 is Monday, Day 2 is Tuesday, Day 3 is Wednesday, Day 4 is Thursday, Day 5 is Friday.

Many new mothers find it helpful to prepare their lunches the evening before, after dinner. Because a mother's morning can be hectic when she's rushing out to work, or to another engagement, it's reassuring to know that your lunch is there waiting for you—one less thing to think about when you're trying to get out of the house. None of the lunches here will suffer from spending a night in the refrigerator, and unless the weather is very hot, they will not require refrigeration for the several hours between your leaving in the morning and lunch hour. (Wrap sandwiches in aluminum foil, then put them in sealable sandwich bags to help them stay cool.)

Recipes

Day 1

VEGGIE SANDWICH
tomato slices
cucumber slices
carrot curls
green pepper rings
lettuce leaves
mustard
1 whole wheat pita bread pocket
2 stalks celery

8-ounce can tomato or V-8 juice
lemon wedge

Day 2

TUNA-CHEESE SANDWICH
1 small can (3¼ oz.) water-packed tuna
1 stick chopped celery
1 slice (1 oz.) part-skim mozzarella, or other low-fat cheese
1 whole wheat pita pocket bread

plain or flavored seltzer or club soda

Day 3

HAM AND CHEESE SANDWICH
1 slice lean ham (about ⅔ oz.)
1 slice (1 oz.) part-skim mozzarella, or other low-fat cheese
tomato slices
mustard
2 thin slices whole wheat or protein bread

plain or flavored seltzer or club soda

Day 4

PRIMAVERA CHEESE SANDWICH
2 slices (1 oz. each) part-skim mozzarella, or other low-fat
    cheese
diced tomato
lettuce leaves
bean sprouts
mustard
1 whole wheat pita bread pocket

plain or flavored seltzer or club soda

Day 5

MIXED BROWN BAG
½ apple, cubed
½ orange, wedges halved
½ banana, sliced
lemon juice
2 slices whole wheat or protein bread or toast

plain or flavored seltzer or club soda

If you prepare fruit the night before, toss the pieces together, spoon into a sealable plastic container, spritz with fresh lemon juice, toss again, and seal the container.

Restaurant Lunches

Many new mothers may find that for business or social reasons, eating lunch in a restaurant is a necessity or an important pleasure. The lunch hour is, of course, a time when many of us do business or fit meetings with friends into our busy schedules.

Eating lunch out may mean grabbing a quick bite in a company cafeteria, or meeting a business associate in an elegant eatery, or catching up with a friend at a casual luncheonette or diner. Because of the wide range of possible lunchtime restaurants, the Post-Pregnancy Diet offers you mix-and-match combinations of foods to make up your noontime meals eaten out. The lists here offer you the choice of one protein dish and two vegetable/fruit portions, with a beverage of your choice. (Coffee and tea, without milk or sugar, are of course, always permitted.)

If you are eating in a luncheonette, diner, or cafeteria, you might put together a meal such as cottage cheese with two slices of dry whole wheat toast, green salad with lemon wedges for dressing, and one apple. In a conventional restaurant, you can always find baked or broiled fish or chicken, green beans or broccoli, and salad with lemon wedges. If your lunchtime companion orders a drink before lunch, you can have club soda with lime or lemon wedge, or tomato juice.

At the beginning of the diet, you may find it helpful to copy these lists on a small index card that you can tuck into your purse or briefcase to take along with you.

Mix-and-Match Selection Charts

Since it is impossible to weigh or measure portion sizes in a restaurant, no quantities are specified on these lists. You will become accustomed to what the Post-Pregnancy Diet portions look like from preparing your evening meals at home, and this will help you to gauge how much of your restaurant portion to eat. Never be reluctant to leave some food on your plate at a restaurant if the portion you are served is too large. And, of course, stop eating as soon as you feel satisfied.

Have One Four- to Six-Ounce Portion from This List

Baked, broiled, steamed, or grilled fish, prepared without butter or sauce
Baked, broiled, or grilled chicken; no butter, no sauce
One broiled or grilled lamb chop
One broiled or grilled veal chop
Baked, broiled, steamed, or boiled shellfish (shrimp, scallops, clams, oysters, lobster, crab); no butter, no sauce
Raw clams or oysters (limit to six)
Cottage cheese with two slices whole wheat bread or dry toast
Two eggs, prepared without fat such as butter or oil

Note: You must remove skin from chicken and trim all visible fat from chops before eating.

Have Two Portions from This List

Green beans
Broccoli
One small baked potato, no butter, dressing, or sour cream
Fresh raw vegetable salad
Green or red pepper
Spinach
Tomato
Carrots
Celery
Squash or zucchini
Cucumber
Onion
Small portion steamed or boiled white or brown rice (half restaurant portion); no butter, no sauce
Bean sprouts
Artichoke (fresh, not marinated or canned in oil)
Asparagus
Brussels sprouts
Cabbage
Radishes
Mushrooms
Fruits (any fresh fruit from Permitted Fruits List)

Note: You may combine any fresh raw vegetables from this list with lettuce to make a fresh salad, which is equivalent to one portion from this list. Order lemon wedges to squeeze over salad greens, or dress with any type of vinegar; steer clear of other dressings.

Restaurant Dinners

Many new mothers find that eating dinner out at a restaurant is an important part of their work and/or social lives. Almost every restaurant will have menu offerings that are compatible with the Post-Pregnancy Diet. You may select a main course from one of the foods on the first list here and have a salad and vegetable with it and fresh fruit for dessert. You may also have a glass of wine with your meal, if you prefer wine to a fruit dessert. As an aperitif you can have tomato or mixed vegetable juice or club soda with a lemon or lime wedge.

One important key to sticking to your diet while dining out is to plan ahead. If you are familiar with the menu you will be choosing from, decide ahead of time what you will be ordering, so only a glance at the choices will be necessary. Menu listings conspire with the atmosphere in a restaurant to stimulate patrons' appetites. You need to have all yours wits about you and keep your willpower in good working order to resist the many temptations you may face. Before you leave for your dinner out, look over the lists here carefully and decide what you will be ordering. Write it down on a small piece of paper you can carry with you.

Rest assured: You *can* enjoy all the pleasures of dining out—having a meal prepared for you and served to you, a pleasant atmosphere for talking with friends or business associates, or time alone with your husband—and stick to your diet, too.

Mix-and-Match Selection Charts

Since it is impossible to weigh or measure portion sizes in a restaurant, no quantities are specified on these lists. You will become accustomed to what the Post-Pregnancy Diet portions look like from preparing your evening meals at home, and this will help you gauge how much of your restaurant portion to eat. Never be reluctant to leave some food on your plate at a restaurant if the portion you are served is too large. And, of course, stop eating as soon as you feel satisfied.

Select One Four- to Six-Ounce Portion from This List

Baked, broiled, steamed, or grilled fish, prepared without
 butter or sauce
Baked, broiled, or grilled chicken or turkey; no butter,
 no sauce
One broiled or grilled lamb chop
One broiled or grilled veal chop
Baked, broiled, steamed, or boiled shellfish (shrimp, scal-
 lops, clams, oysters, lobster, crab); no butter, no sauce
Raw clams or oysters (limit to six)
Baked or roasted turkey, no gravy
One small broiled or grilled steak

Note: You must remove skin from chicken or turkey and trim all visible fat from chops or steak before eating.

Note: No dressing on salad. Order lemon wedges to spritz over salad, or use any type of vinegar, plus one tablespoon of oil, preferably corn oil. (Use a soup spoon or two teaspoons to measure oil for salad at table. Many dieters who dine out frequently carry their own corn oil with them in purse-sized, very leakproof bottles, such as the small plastic travel bottles usually used for toiletries.)

Have a Salad Made of Any
or All of the Following Raw Vegetables

Lettuce
Tomato
Cucumber
Onion
Scallion
Green pepper
Mushrooms
Radishes
Spinach
Carrots
Celery
Bean sprouts

Select One Vegetable from This List

One small baked potato; no butter, no dressing, or sour
   cream
One small portion steamed or boiled white or brown rice
   (half restaurant portion); no butter, no sauce
Squash, zucchini, broccoli, or green beans, steamed or
   boiled
Asparagus; no butter or sauce
Artichoke; no butter, no dressing

You May Also Have

One glass of red or white dry table wine
or
One serving of fresh fruit from Permitted Fruits List

Chapter 3

⌒

Guidelines for
Nursing Mothers

Nursing mothers who wish to control their weight while breast-feeding may follow the Post-Pregnancy Diet, adding a few supplements to increase calories and nutritional values to the necessary levels. The amount of calories each woman may require to maintain a healthy milk supply and to prevent nutritional depletion of her own body varies from one individual to another; 500 to 600 extra calories per day is considered the norm. Also, breast-feeding moms need to increase their milk intake and the amount of protein they consume daily.

Following the Post-Pregnancy Diet with the special additions for nursing mothers solves all the nutritional and caloric equations for you. These supplements will up the diet's daily calories by the required 500 to 600 and increase your calcium and protein intake to a healthy level for nursing. Best of all, the very tasty and filling extras for breast-feeders do not add sugar or unhealthy fats to your diet, and this can help you establish the long-term wholesome eating habits that make lifetime weight control easy and healthful.

The special supplements for nursing mothers include ten "Snacks for Breast-feeding Moms"—a new and different, utterly delicious snack for every day of your diet program—plus two New Mom's Milkshakes each day. Adding extra calories and nutrients to the diet in this way allows you to tailor your eating program to your own needs and wishes.

Show the Post-Pregnancy Diet, with "Guidelines for Nursing Mothers," to your obstetrician or health care practitioner, and discuss with him the individual health needs of you and your baby, as well as your personal diet goals. Each snack represents about 300 calories; each New Mom's Milkshake provides about 150 calories; one snack plus two milkshakes daily supply the nutritional extras you need as well as the additional 500 to 600+ calories. But, in conjunction with your medical professional, you may decide to adjust the number of snacks and milkshakes you have each day in order to increase or decrease daily caloric and/or nutritional intake. Several combinations are possible for meeting your own needs and goals. Many nursing mothers will find that the best course to take is to begin the diet with guidelines as it is specified here and, if necessary, adjust the eating plan and supplements in accordance with how well the program works for you.

The Post-Pregnancy Diet with "Guidelines for Nursing Mothers" is based on established averages of nutritional and caloric needs. It will help most breast-feeding women supply plenty of milk for their babies, meet their own bodies' needs, and control their weight. It is designed to be flexible, however, so that you can adjust your intake according to your individual needs. Best of all, as you begin weaning your baby, and your caloric needs are accordingly reduced, you can start to cut back on snacks gradually. By the time you've stopped breast-feeding, you can begin dieting without the extra snacks—and you'll be way ahead of the game, having already lost some of the weight you want to take off.

Supplemental Snacks for Breast-Feeding Moms

Follow the Post-Pregnancy Diet five-day eating plans as specified on the preceding pages, and add to your daily meal schedules:

- Two New Mom's Milkshakes (one at mid-morning, the other before bed)
  plus

- One of the following mid-afternoon snacks

Crunchy Date Delight

½ cup plain low-fat yogurt
¼ cup whole grain cereal or granola (check the label to be sure no sugars or honey have been added)
¼ cup chopped dates

Mix together.

Pea Soup Snack

1 cup split pea soup
2 tablespoons grated parmesan cheese

Sprinkle cheese on top of soup.

"Cheese Cake"

1 brown rice cake
4 tablespoons part-skim mozzarella cheese, shredded

Top rice cake with mozzarella. Broil for 3 minutes.

Shrimp Boat

1 cup cream of shrimp soup prepared with skim milk
¼ lb. boiled baby shrimp

Sprinkle shrimp on top of soup.

Pita Jelly Fruit Roll

1 whole wheat pita pocket bread
2 tablespoons low-fat cottage cheese
4 strawberries, sliced
2 tablespoons fruit-juice-sweetened jam or jelly

Toast pita. Mix remaining ingredients together and fill pita pocket with mixture.

Pop Munch

¼ cup raisins
1 cup popcorn (popped in hot-air popper)

Mix raisins and popcorn.

Clam Chowder

1 cup New England-style clam chowder prepared with skim milk
"croutons" (1 slice whole wheat or protein bread, toasted, cut 3 times lengthwise, 3 times crosswise to make 9 cubes)

Sprinkle "croutons" on top of soup.

Tropicana Treat

½ fresh pear, cubed
1 tangerine, sectioned, with sections cut in half
1 tablespoon shredded coconut

Toss together pear cubes and tangerine sections. Sprinkle
with coconut.

Mushroom Mug

1 cup cream of mushroom soup prepared with skim milk
1 tablespoon dried chives

Sprinkle chives on top of soup.

Spiced "Banana Cake"

1 brown rice cake
3 tablespoons low-fat cottage cheese
½ banana, sliced
sprinkling of cinnamon

Spread cottage cheese on rice cake. Top with banana and
sprinkle with cinnamon.

Chapter 4

⌒

Weekend Strategies and Forbidden Foods

The Post-Pregnancy Diet is designed to make life as easy as possible for new moms, and having "diet-free" weekends is an important part of that plan. On Saturday and Sunday, you don't have to stick to the exact salad-for-lunch-chicken-for-dinner meal plans that you must follow the rest of the week. This gives you more freedom to vary your eating patterns (have a big breakfast, a late lunch, and a small snack in the evening, for example), even to go out to eat at a friend's house.

But having weekends off also means you have to take more responsibility for yourself and your eating. You'll find that the Post-Pregnancy Diet does most of the work for you Monday through Friday. On weekends, you'll be practicing the diet skills you learn during the week, but you'll have to create your own format and rely more on your ability to control your eating.

You already know that you are not allowed any sugars or fats during your "diet-free" weekends, and if you are in doubt about a specific food, make sure it's not on the list of "Forbidden Fat and Sugar Foods" on p. 97. What you'll want to explore and focus on over the weekend are those foods you *can* enjoy, as well as new techniques for making this diet a part of your everyday life. Refer back to the "Permitted Ingredients for Dinner Preparation" list in the previous chapter (p. 44) to get ideas for new ways to prepare your weekend meals. Here are some more tips for your "diet-free" weekend.

"Diet-Free" Breakfast, Lunch, and Dinner

Planning your own meals on Saturdays and Sundays may give you a wonderful sense of freedom, or it may make you feel uncertain about your ability to stick to the diet without the structure of exact meal plans. If you are worried about how to handle your weekends at first you might want to use your favorite meal plans from the week for Saturday and Sunday meals. Just pick out your favorite breakfasts, lunches, and dinners, and follow those menus over the weekend until you are farther along on the diet and feel more confident in your ability to create your own diet with no sugar or fat.

Once you feel comfortable making your own choices on the weekend, you can enjoy some spontaneity with meals if you make sure to prepare your household, and specifically your kitchen, beforehand. The two most important elements of preparing for your Post-Pregnancy Diet weekends are:

• Make sure there aren't any forbidden food temptations in your kitchen over the weekend. If other family members have favorite foods that fall into the sugar or fat category, ask that they not store and eat those foods at home over the weekend, or at least that these foods be kept in one out-of-the-way place where you won't see them and be tempted by them.

• Stock your kitchen with plenty of foods you *can* eat. Go to your supermarket toward the end of the week, or on Saturday morning, armed with your list of permitted food, and buy everything that strikes your fancy. You will find that fresh fruits and vegetables, pasta of every variety, full-flavored whole-grain breads and crackers, fresh, light-tasting, low-fat cottage cheese and yogurt, and lean meats, poultry, and fish are very appealing choices.

Some dieters will find that they prefer to create meal plans before the "diet-free" weekend to make sure there are no surprises and nothing is left to chance. If you will feel more at ease knowing exactly what you will be eating on Saturday and Sunday, it's a good idea to sit down Friday evening or Saturday morning and make up your own meal plans for the weekend. You can use some of the menus you like from the weekday meal plans, create your own menus, or use some of the weekend recipes included here (see p. 92).

When you become more confident of your ability to stick to the diet and at the same time indulge your food whims of the moment, you will really start to appreciate all the freedom you have over the weekend on the Post-Pregnancy Diet. Weekends provide time when new moms should enjoy the pleasures of unstructured time and a respite from the demands of weekday schedules. Taking a break from your diet seems to fit right into this mood, and it will work if you are very strict about avoiding sugar and fat foods. Here are some specific strategies for meals.

Breakfast

No new mother should deny herself the luxury of big morning meals on Saturday and Sunday. You may not be able to partake of some of the more typical indulgences, which shall go unmentioned here, but you can create a "groaning board" of fresh fruit cut into serving size, a bowl of low-fat yogurt with ground cinnamon and vanilla extract stirred in, as a dip for your fruit, whole wheat (and sugarless, of course) bread and crackers spread with low-fat cottage cheese and sprinkled with fresh herbs, favorite vegetables cut into chunks for a crudité platter, even broiled fish fillet with lemon juice and fresh herbs.

It's especially pleasant to prepare a big breakfast spread that the whole family can enjoy, including the toddler who likes finger foods. And, if the breakfast foods are wholesome, filling, and low in calories, a large morning meal can be the start to a good diet day, because you'll burn off breakfast calories more efficiently than the calories consumed later in the day.

When weekend morning plans include trying to get to a playdate, or puppet show, or anything else on time, and your breakfast is more hurried, there are several quick-take morning foods to enjoy. Whole wheat toast spread with low-fat cottage cheese and topped with banana slices is delicious and filling. A melon wedge filled with low-fat cottage cheese is quick and tasty. Do try to keep in mind, however, that when you have to prepare food in a hurry, it will satisfy best if you can eat it as slowly as possible. Even a hurry-up breakfast will feel more filling for a longer time when you take at least ten minutes to sit down and eat it slowly.

Lunch

Weekend lunches can vary from a quick bite between activities to the big family meal of the day. The plans you make, the shape the day takes on, and your own appetite are the guides you'll use in determining what kind of lunch is right on a given Saturday or Sunday. The weekend recipes included in this section are great for lunch fare, or you may find simple sandwiches more appropriate.

One new mother found it helpful to roast a large chicken or turkey on Saturday morning, make a big meal of it for Saturday lunch, toss it in with a green salad for Saturday dinner, and have sandwiches on Sunday. (If you decide to follow her example, remove all skin from your portion.)

Even though you can eat as much as you like on "diet-free" weekends, you might find yourself the least hungry at lunchtime on those days when you have a big breakfast and plans for a big dinner. On such days, your New Mom's Milkshake or one of the supplemental snacks for nursing mothers may be just right for you at midday. Don't feel you have to eat a full meal just because it's mealtime. Pay close attention to your own appetite, and eat only as much as you are hungry for.

Dinner

The evening meal on the weekend might be anything from a quick bite before the movies on a precious evening out, to having company over for a big Saturday night supper. Because the Post-Pregnancy Diet gives you "diet-free" weekends, you can have this kind of flexibility with your dinners.

If you like to be creative in the kitchen, weekends are a wonderful time to experiment with the new no-sugar, no-fat approach to cooking you've been using all week with your diet menus. On a Saturday or Sunday evening, you're likely to have more time to spend enjoying meal preparation, and it's a good time to try adding some different herbs, or any of the other permitted ingredients, to your diet dishes.

I think you'll find that you can cook for company quite easily within the guidelines of the Post-Pregnancy Diet. Many people these days are rather conscious of what they eat and prefer the lighter style of food preparation that minimizes the use of fats. Keep in mind that you are allowed one tablespoon of corn oil or corn oil margarine per day, so a recipe that serves several people and calls for no more than one tablespoon of oil or margarine per serving is perfectly permissible.

Also keep in mind that you are allowed a glass of wine with your evening meal, so you won't have to feel deprived if you serve your company wine at dinner. If a guest asks if she can bring something, suggest she bring a dessert. This provides something sweet for those who want it, and means that you'll have minimal contact with high-calorie desserts you can offer to your guests. And *always* serve a big bowl of attractive fruits at the end of your dinners, so you'll have something tasty to chew when the meal is over.

Look through your favorite recipe books and see if there are some good recipes you can adapt to your new style of cooking and eating. I think you'll find that many good recipes need be modified only slightly to fit into your "diet-free" weekend. Here are some simple techniques that will help you turn a standard recipe into a Post-Pregnancy Diet recipe:

- Remove skin from poultry, and all visible fat from meat.

- Try substituting low-fat yogurt when recipes call for sour cream, heavy cream, or mayonnaise.

- Use corn oil margarine (no more than one tablespoon per serving, per day) instead of butter; use corn oil (one tablespoon per serving per day) instead of other oils.

- Try substituting two egg whites for each whole egg specified in a recipe.

- Make your own bread crumbs from whole-grain breads, toasted and grated, or crushed with a rolling pin.

As you experiment with cooking the Post-Pregnancy Diet way, you'll probably find other ways to make changes in your cooking techniques so that you can still enjoy preparing and eating delicious food, without the unhealthy sugar and fat, without the extra calories, but with plenty of good nourishment for yourself and your entire family.

Entertainments

Before long you will probably feel quite secure with your weekend freedom, and you will know just how to handle all your Saturday and Sunday meals. If you have company for a meal, you'll be able to serve good-tasting food and still stick to your diet. If you eat out in a restaurant, you can follow the guidelines given for following the diet in a restaurant. The only kind of socializing that could present a problem for you is being a dinner guest at a friend's home.

It's always difficult to stick to a diet when you're invited to dinner. This diet provides you with the flexibility of a weekend off from scheduled meals, however, and that should help. There are specific strategies as well, depending on the situation.

If you are invited to dinner at the home of a close friend, you might feel quite comfortable telling your friend that you're dieting and asking what she or he is planning to serve, so that you can plan ahead a bit. You can eat most everyday foods if you trim fat from meat, skin from poultry, avoid rich sauces, and don't add butter or oily dressings to vegetables or salads. These are techniques you can employ inconspicuously at any dinner table, and the more familiar you become with them, the more routinely you can use them to your diet advantage at a dinner party.

But, then, of course, there's always the possibility that you won't feel comfortable calling your hosts in advance, and you'll arrive at dinner only to find you're being served a heaping helping of lasagna. In such situations, your first tactic should be to try to have as little of the food as possible on your plate. (Even when confronted with lasagna, you can try to eat mostly the pasta and as little as possible of the oily sauce and high-fat cheese.) Ask for a small helping, or take a small helping if you can serve yourself at a buffet.

Even if you get stuck at a dinner table with a fattening and forbidden main course, you needn't go hungry if you can fill up on other side dishes—vegetables, salad,* even bread with no butter. Do your best to have as little as possible (or none at all, if you can) of the food not on your diet without being too obvious about it. Keep in mind that your diet is one of your top priorities at this point, and it's worth the extra concentration you'll need to apply on certain social occasions to stay on your path to your pre-pregnancy figure.

If you're going to slip up on your diet, it's most likely to happen in a social situation such as a dinner party. You could end up having to take a few bites of a food you shouldn't be eating, and that really doesn't have to be so terrible. Just get right back on your diet, without dwelling on the incident.

Use all the good diet strategies you know to keep yourself on your diet: While others sip cocktails before dinner, have a big glass of club soda, seltzer, or plain water to fill yourself up. Eat slowly so that you're aware of each mouthful; chew each bite for a long time before you take the next one; think about everything you put into your mouth, mentally checking to make sure that the food has no fat or sugar. On the Post-Pregnancy Diet, you only have two rules to remember—no fat, no sugar—and that should help make your eating choices as simple as they can be, no matter what the situation.

Staying in the Diet Mode

By the time you arrive at your first "weekend off, with guidelines," you will have followed a schedule of three healthful, low-calorie, high-nutrient meals a day, with only your milkshake or the special supplements for nursing

---

*Salads will probably have an oil-based dressing, so your salad serving will include your one-tablespoon-of-corn-oil allowance for the day.

moms, as a snack. After the very first week of dieting, you are bound to be in "the dieting mode," psyched-up to stick to your diet, already losing weight and feeling lighter and thinner, and highly motivated to make the diet work for you until you arrive at your goal.

On your first five days on the Post-Pregnancy Diet, I think you will find that your eating habits are already changing, and much more easily than you might have believed possible. Cravings for sugary and/or fatty foods have probably diminished or vanished altogether; your appetite in general is apt to be reduced; smaller portions of most foods tend to feel more satisfying; and temptations to eat between meals have usually faded, or at least been channeled into an appetite for the refreshing New Mom's Shake, or the wholesome, nonfattening foods included among the supplemental snacks for nursing mothers. You will be better prepared than you might think to stick to a less structured diet of no sugar, no fat. And, in many cases, you will probably discover that you can continue to lose weight over your "diet-free" weekend.

If you find, however, that you don't lose, but only maintain your weight over the weekend, or if you gain a tiny bit, you will need to review your eating for the weekend. First, make sure there are no hidden sugars or fats in the foods you are eating. Check labels on prepared foods, and double-check the list of forbidden foods. If that doesn't seem to be the problem, you will have to cut back on quantity a bit. Protein foods (meat or poultry, for example) and complex carbohydrates like whole grains, rice, and pasta are the most calorie-dense of the foods you are permitted on this diet, and you may have to eat less of these.

Usually, when there are weekend gains on this diet, you can discover and isolate the culprit(s), and eliminate the problems the following weekend, after another week of consistent weight losses on the formal program. Don't become frustrated if you're not losing as quickly over the weekends at first. You will definitely start losing again the following Monday, and the longer you stay on the diet, the more easily you will lose on the weekends.

Your "diet-free" weekends are like training periods for the eating style you will want to practice when you have arrived at your goal weight and completed the formal diet. As such, they provide you with an opportunity to discover new ways of enjoying food without the constrictions of a diet, and without gaining weight. Use your "diet-free" weekends to be good to yourself, and to learn as much as you can about adapting your personal eating style to the guidelines of no sugar, no fats.

Weekend Recipes

I think weekend meals are different from workaday meals. Saturdays and Sundays not only allow you more time for food preparation, they also lend themselves to a different and more leisurely style of eating. The weekend recipes included here—a soup, a pasta dish, and a salad—are each meals in themselves, dishes you can prepare for Saturday lunch and enjoy for Sunday meals as well. Recipes serve six to eight, depending on portion size, and leftovers may be saved for later meals.

Recipes

Salmon/Clam Chowder
(serves 6 to 8)

2 tablespoons corn oil
1 medium onion, chopped
1 small green pepper, chopped
2 medium potatoes, peeled and diced
1 large carrot, pared and sliced
1 large stalk celery, sliced
4 cups water
1 bay leaf
⅛ teaspoon pepper
¼ teaspoon thyme
2 teaspoons dill seed
2 tablespoons uncooked rice
1 16-ounce can whole tomatoes in tomato juice
1 6½-ounce can pink salmon, with liquid
1 6½-ounce can minced clams, with liquid
(or substitute ¾ pound fresh fish or shellfish for canned
  salmon and clams)

Heat corn oil over medium heat in a large, heavy pot
with cover; add chopped onion and pepper; sauté five
minutes. Add potatoes, carrot, and celery; continue cooking for another five minutes. Add water, seasonings,
rice, and tomatoes. Reduce heat to simmer. Stir tomatoes, breaking up large pieces with the back of the spoon.
Simmer thirty minutes, covered. Add fresh or canned
fish, heat through, and serve immediately.

May be stored in the refrigerator for two or three days
and reheated to serve; may be frozen for several weeks.

Fettucine Primavera
(serves 6 to 8)

2 tablespoons corn oil
½ pound mushrooms, cleaned and sliced
1 clove garlic, minced fine
4 scallions, both white and green parts, chopped
1 red pepper, cut into thin strips
1 teaspoon oregano
2 cups plain, low-fat yogurt
1 egg white, beaten foamy
⅛ cup grated parmesan cheese
1 pound whole wheat, spinach, or plain fettucine, or other
shape pasta

Heat corn oil over medium heat in a large, deep skillet.
Add mushrooms, garlic, and scallions; sauté five minutes, stirring often. Add red pepper strips, continue cooking two minutes more. Add oregano to vegetables.
Combine yogurt, egg white, and cheese in a medium
bowl; add to skillet. Reduce heat to lowest setting and
heat through, stirring constantly, about three minutes.
Do *not* allow mixture to boil. Cook fettucine or pasta to *al
dente* stage following package directions; drain and trans-
fer to warmed bowl. Add vegetable/yogurt sauce and toss
well. Serve immediately.

May be stored in the refrigerator for three days and
served chilled or reheated.

Salad Dijonnaise
(serves 6 to 8)

5 cups lettuce, any type, torn into bite-size pieces
4 large tomatoes, quartered, quarters cut in half
or
6 plum tomatoes, quartered
or
1 pint cherry tomatoes, halved
1 cucumber, scrubbed, cut in half lengthwise, and sliced
1 small red onion, sliced thin
2 cups mushrooms, cleaned and sliced
1 green pepper, scrubbed and seeded, sliced into rings
2 cups cooked chicken, cubed or julienned
1 cup part-skim mozzarella or other low-fat cheese, cubed
   or julienned

Toss vegetables together in large bowl. Serve dressing (recipe follows) on the side. Salad may be covered tightly to store in refrigerator for two days if dressing is not added to salad bowl.

Dijonnaise Dressing

(Makes enough for generous five to six tablespoons of dressing for each large serving of salad recipe)

2 cups plain low-fat yogurt
3 tablespoons Dijon mustard
2 tablespoons lemon juice
1 tablespoon grated lemon rind
3 tablespoons finely minced parsley
1 clove garlic, pressed

Use a whisk to beat together yogurt, mustard, and lemon juice in a small bowl. Stir in lemon rind and parsley. Use garlic press to press garlic clove into mixture; stir to combine. Store covered in refrigerator. May be stored three to four days; garlic will become stronger.

Forbidden Foods

Following are lists of most of the foods that fall into the two forbidden categories on the Post-Pregnancy Diet: fats and sugars. If you are in doubt about a food containing fat, and you do not find it on the list here, it is best not to eat it until you can look it up in a reference that lists the amounts of fat in given foods. Items that you suspect contain sugar probably do. When in doubt, don't eat the food in question. Most prepared foods will list the amount of fat and sugar contained in the food on the package or label of the product. Avoid products that list any form of sugar in the ingredients and that contain more than five grams of fat per serving.

During the week, your diet menu plans include one tablespoon of corn oil or one tablespoon of corn oil margarine each day. You'll want to include the same amount in your daily diet on weekends as well. This provides a healthy amount of fat in a wholesome form recommended by nutritionists. You may also have certain low-fat dairy products in unlimited amounts over the weekend—low-fat yogurt and low-fat cottage cheese offer protein, some calcium, and other important nutrients. You can drink as much reconstituted nonfat dry milk as you like. And, to add taste and increase calcium a bit more, you may have limited daily amounts of three more dairy foods as follows:

- One ounce low-fat or part-skim cheese

- One tablespoon grated hard cheese (parmesan or romano)

• Half a cup (four ounces) skim milk

You'll want to look over the lists that follow before the weekend begins, and you will probably need to refer back to the lists at times to make sure you are not including any of the listed foods in your weekend menus. But do try to focus on those foods you *can* enjoy. Weekends are a time when you can be free from the usual constraints and pressures of weekday schedules and set meal plans, so you'll want to think positive and find new ways to prepare and appreciate the permitted foods.

Note: As explained in the introduction to this book, it's difficult to have "diet alternative" foods on hand—sugar substitutes, commercially prepared diet mayonnaise or salad dressing, sugar-free cookies and candies—when you have a toddler around who wants to eat everything you eat. Even if your child is much too young to be interested in your food, you won't want to get in the habit of relying on "diet" foods that you won't be able to share with your child later. One of the advantages of this diet for new mothers is that all the wholesome, natural foods included in the diet are good for your children and your entire family; your diet will never have to involve making separate dishes for yourself at family meal times. For this reason, diet foods are not included on the Post-Pregnancy Diet. This is a diet that will show you how to eliminate sugar and reduce the amount of fat and calories you consume, without relying on diet foods with all their chemical additives.

Also, as I explain in the next chapter, fruit juices can become a high-calorie habit for nursing mothers, one that persists even after your child has been weaned. You can eat all the filling, tasty fresh fruits you want over the weekend, but you have to give up all fruit juices, even though they do not fall into the category either of fats or sugars. Whole fruits offer more of the same nutrients than juices do—and at far fewer calories.

And, remember, your four-ounce glass of wine *with* your dinner (not before, since it may stimulate your appetite on an empty stomach) is the only alcoholic beverage you are allowed on this diet, during the week and over the weekend. (You may, however, use two ounces of dry table wine as a cooking ingredient if you wish, as specified in "Permitted Ingredients for Dinner Preparation," p. 44.)

The Forbidden Fats

- All oil and margarine, except one tablespoon corn oil or one tablespoon corn oil margarine daily
- All cheese, except one ounce low-fat or part-skim cheese, plus one tablespoon grated hard cheese (parmesan, romano) daily
- All milk, except half a cup of skim milk daily, plus as much nonfat dry milk (reconstituted) as desired
- Fried foods
- All chips (potato, corn, tortilla, banana)
- Bacon
- Butter
- Cream cheese
- Mayonnaise
- Nuts and nut butters
- Fast food hamburgers, fish fillets, fried chicken, french fries
- Sour cream, heavy cream, half-and-half
- Egg yolk
- Olives

- Avocado

- Popcorn (unless hot-air popped)

- Frankfurters, liverwurst, knockwurst, bratwurst, kielbasa

- Salami, pepperoni, all sausages, prosciutto

- Bologna, all luncheon meats

- Cheese spreads and cheese foods

- Hollandaise sauce

- Croissant, puff pastry, piecrust

- Ice cream, malteds, milkshakes, ice cream sodas

- Lard, shortening

- Mexican foods: refried beans, tacos, tostadas, enchiladas, tamales, quesadillas, burritos

- Chinese foods: egg roll, fried rice, sweet and sour dishes, all fried foods and foods prepared with oil

- Tempura vegetables or seafood

- Oil or dry roasted sunflower nuts and sunflower seeds

- Sesame butter, sesame paste, tahini

- Blintzes

- Tartar sauce

- Gravy

- Smoked fish

- All fish packed or canned in oil

- Corned beef

- Pastrami

- Paté

- Pork rinds
- Unsweetened chocolate
- Batter-dipped or breaded frozen fish, or chicken
- Fritters, hush puppies
- Croutons
- Pizza
- Spaghetti sauces, chili (you may make your own however, using lean meat and one tablespoon corn oil per serving)
- Commercially prepared dips and salad dressings
- Hashed brown potatoes, home fries
- Visible fat on meat
- Poultry skin

The Forbidden Sugars

- All sugar (white, brown, refined, raw)
- All sweeteners in prepared foods, such as sucrose, lactose, fructose, corn sweeteners, dextrose
- Honey
- Molasses
- Corn syrup
- Cookies
- Candy
- Cake
- Doughnuts, sweet rolls, muffins, raisin bread
- Jams, jellies, preserves (except those sweetened with fruit juice)

- Soda (except seltzer, club soda)
- Catsup
- Barbecue sauce
- Worcestershire or other steak sauces
- Sweet pickles or relishes
- Mustards prepared with sugar or honey
- Pies
- Pudding
- Gelatin desserts or salads
- Ice milk, frozen yogurt, sherbet, fruit ices, frozen fruit bars
- Fruit yogurt, flavored yogurt
- Cole slaw
- Pancakes, waffles, french toast
- Maple syrup, maple-flavored syrup
- All chocolate products
- Canned fruits
- Fruit rolls
- Dried fruits
- Baked beans
- Granola bars, breakfast bars
- Date-nut bread, banana bread, zucchini bread, carrot cake
- Brownies
- Sweetened applesauce
- Chewing gum, breath mints

Chapter 5

◦—

The Stages-of-Motherhood Guide to the Diet

Your ability to stick to a good weight-loss program is always influenced by the way you live, your work and social schedules, your feelings of satisfaction and fulfillment, your moods and attitudes. All these elements of lifestyle are profoundly affected by the new member of your family, and of course, as soon as you feel certain that you and the baby have finally established a routine, the baby is apt to change again. As babies and young children follow the natural course of early development, they seem to be in constant change, and because every diet requires a certain amount of foresight and planning, your ever-changing life as a new mother can sometimes prove frustrating.

The overall key to success in sustaining a diet throughout your early motherhood is to anticipate the inevitable changes in routine that your baby will bring. I think you'll find that with all you have to do and all you have to think about during this time, the Post-Pregnancy Diet will really help you eat healthfully and lose weight without much extra effort on your part. Here's some additional guidance to help you through some of the rough spots.

From Your Child's Birth to Three Months

This is a phase of new motherhood that varies greatly from one woman to the next. For some, there is a euphoric high, a complete and exclusive focus on the baby. For others, the first three months are a nightmare of sleepless nights, constant fatigue and frustration, insecurity, and confusion. And for everyone, there are changes that will affect your ability to care for yourself, as well as your baby.

Breast-feeding

If you are nursing your infant, this is the time when the baby is apt to be consuming a great deal of nourishment from your body. Some women feel very hungry during the time they breast-feed—even hungrier than they did while pregnant. Almost everyone feels very thirsty. Some nursing mothers become reliant on fruit juices at this time, and several have reported that it was difficult to give up juice when they went on the Post-Pregnancy Diet.

There is a very definite reason why no fruit juices are included in this diet: Although juice is a healthful and wholesome drink, it lacks some important elements that you derive from eating the whole fruit. Some nutrients and most of the fiber of a fruit are left behind when the juice is extracted—and, most important to dieters, the calories in fruit juice are almost double the amount in the whole fruit. Half a grapefruit has about 50 calories; an eight-ounce glass of grapefruit juice has just over 100 calories. A whole orange has about 65 calories; an eight-ounce glass of orange juice has about 120 calories.

There's plenty of whole fruit included in the Post-Pregnancy Diet; you eat fruit for breakfast every day, sometimes at lunch, in your New Mom's Milkshake, and often at dinner. You get all the vitamins, nutrients, and fiber you need from the fruit you eat on this diet, and the fruits themselves are a more complete and filling source of this essential nourishment than juices are. Juice is a tasty drink for new mothers, but unfortunately, it is too fattening to be included in a good weight-loss program for recent moms who want to lose weight.

Also, water is a better thirst-quencher. Pure, plain water from the tap, spring water, mineral water, club soda, and seltzer tend to hydrate your system more quickly, and satisfy your thirst better. If you have become accustomed to settling down to breast-feed with a tall glass of juice by your side, switch to an inviting glass of your favorite kind of water. Add some ice and a wedge of lemon or lime, or try one of the flavored seltzers. Drink as much water as you want and need.

I know of two women who gained upward of ten pounds during the first three months of nursing. Both were mystified about their weight gains because they were eating normally and being careful about avoiding fats and sweets. When I asked them to keep track of how much juice they drank, they each reported about eight to ten glasses a day, which they drank while nursing. They were shocked to learn that they were adding 900 to 1,200 calories to their daily calorie count just by drinking juice! Thirsty breast-feeding moms can easily forget that what they drink may have even more calories than what they eat. This diet will help you switch to eating fruit and drinking water.

The Post-Pregnancy Diet allows you to eat to match your appetite, so if you are one of those breast-feeding mothers who feels ravenously hungry, you can fill up on the "Supplemental Snacks for Breast-feeding Moms." In these early stages of nursing, you may feel the need to have two New Mom's Milkshakes and two snacks, in addition to your three meals, a day. You don't have to deny your hunger on this diet, but do try to stay in touch with your body's real needs. If you start to supplement your breast milk with formula, and your baby is drinking less of your milk, you are apt to feel less hungry, and it may be time to eliminate some of your daily snacks. Adjust your snacks to your appetite, but before you eat anything, always stop to ask yourself if you really are hungry. There may be times when you feel depleted and thirsty, and a glass of water, plus a short, refreshing catnap will satisfy you just as well as something to eat.

Meal Scheduling

The very idea of eating three normal meals at approximately the normal meal hours can seem like an impossible goal to the mother of a six-week-old baby. Some new moms report that they can hardly keep track of the day of the week, let alone the hour of the day, during this period of very erratic sleeping hours and near constant demands from the baby. Nonetheless, trying to establish some semblance of regular eating hours is one of the best ways possible to start getting back to normal. Even if you can't have breakfast at eight, lunch at noon, and dinner at six every night, approximating a regular meal schedule is one of the best things a new mother can do to make herself feel like part of the human race again.

At this early stage of mothering, you needn't put undue pressure on yourself to eat each of your meals at exactly the time that the rest of the world is probably having that meal. There will be many times that the usual breakfast, lunch, or dinner hours are the times of day for you to get some much-needed sleep, do the laundry, or run errands. But do try to get into the habit of spacing your meals about four or five hours apart.

Take each day as it comes. If your day with the baby starts at 5 A.M., have breakfast then, lunch at 11, your New Mom's Milkshake at 2 P.M., dinner at 5. If the baby sleeps off and on until 10 one morning, and you can sleep, too, get your rest, then have a late breakfast at 10, lunch at 3, dinner at 7.

If you're breast-feeding and are eating Supplemental Snacks, keep them as evenly spaced as possible between meals, having your snacks at least two hours after the last meal and two hours before the next meal.

As long as the new baby's routine is erratic and change-able, you may not be able to schedule your own day exactly as you would like it, but you can control the spacing of meals and snacks, even if you can't always plan for the right hours of the day for meals. Getting your body accustomed to regular intervals between meals is excellent behavior training that will help you adjust your eating habits to a more healthful and slimming regime.

New mothers who are at home most of the day for the first time may be overwhelmed by the temptation to nibble throughout the day or grab a bite here and there when they get the chance. The Post-Pregnancy Diet will help all new mothers become attuned to a regular eating schedule, even if it's not at the usual hours of the day, and this will prove very helpful to long-term weight loss.

As much as possible, take time to have your meals and snacks. No matter what the hour of day that you're having a meal, try to allow for some unharried time to prepare and eat your food. Meal preparation on the Post-Pregnancy Diet requires a minimal amount of time, but you should allow yourself at least a half hour to sit down at a table and really enjoy your food. Think of your meals as times of day when you do something nice for yourself by preparing and enjoying healthful, wholesome, low-calorie food that helps you take off the weight you gained during pregnancy.

Fatigue

During the first three months of new motherhood, being tired can become a way of life. Sleep deprivation affects your body in several ways, and it can make you feel depleted and depressed. If you tend to overeat when you feel down, your mood during this period can certainly jeopardize your diet. Feelings of depletion can also cause you to overeat, because food provides a quick pickup when energy flags. Making an effort to avoid excess fatigue will be an important part of your dieting success.

One of the most common diet traps for mothers of infants is eating when they really need sleep. There are many times when you need sleep but you just can't get it—because the baby is awake and needs you, because you have chores to finish, because other family members need you or you need them. Often, when you feel exhausted but you can't take a nap, there is a temptation to fill up on food to make yourself feel better.

For your overall well-being and health, you must focus on getting plenty of rest and sleep during the first three months of mothering. Food may make you feel better temporarily when you're very, very tired, but it won't really help your body's craving for rest. Make sleep a top priority for yourself, and try not to let other obligations interfere with your getting all the rest you need. You already know from your own experience all the reasons that sleep is so important to you now—fatigue affects your mood, energy level, patience, and attitude, to name but a few. In addition, a lack of sleep can really affect your ability to stay on a diet.

In my family, we have a saying that goes, "When tired, eat; when hungry, sleep." I was often reminded of this nonsense phrase during my baby's first three months of life. At 3 A.M., after nursing her, I'd find myself sleep-walking down to the kitchen for a snack, and in the early evening, just after the baby had fallen asleep, I'd plan to start making dinner, then fall asleep on the couch instead. All new mothers will have times like these, but the best advice possible is to stay in touch with your body's real needs. When you're tired, get some sleep, or at least some rest, even if it means getting help from friends or relatives or hiring help. And, when you're hungry, enjoy your Post-Pregnancy Diet meals, or the supplement snacks for nursing mothers. Try to keep fatigue and hunger separate by concentrating on what your body really needs at any given time.

Your Own Time

Almost every diet recommends that you take the time to be good to yourself—in some way other than eating—while you're on a diet. Treating yourself well boosts your morale and helps you explore the possibility of nonedible treats and rewards. Taking time to yourself while you're on this special diet is *essential*. You'll have strict priorities during the first three months of motherhood: Your baby's needs will probably come first, your own needs for rest and good nutrition should come next, and for a healthy state of mind, taking time to yourself is an excellent third priority. With so many demands on your time and energy, your psychological well-being and your ability to care for yourself by eating well and losing the extra pregnancy weight may be strongly influenced by simply giving yourself your own time.

Start by giving yourself a reasonable amount of time to prepare and enjoy your meals and snacks. Try very hard to eat only when your baby is sleeping or resting quietly and not in need of your attention. Gulping down some nourishment and trying to comfort or care for an infant at the same time is neither satisfying to your hunger nor fulfilling to your needs to nourish yourself. Take time to eat so you can focus on enjoying your food. And, as much as possible, create a calm and comfortable atmosphere for yourself so you can concentrate on eating. This can make an enormous difference in your ability to gain satisfaction from the food you eat and to learn to control your eating behavior.

Also, to the greatest extent possible, plan pleasant things to do that are self-nurturing and *don't* involve eating. Some mothers report this is a difficult assignment, both because it may be hard to plan ahead and because so often you feel that your time is no longer your own. It can be very helpful to your dieting efforts, however, to appreciate yourself as an individual apart from your baby. Many new mothers have reported that they hardly noticed how fat they were during the period they were relatively homebound, spending most of their time with the new baby. Hiring a babysitter, or asking for help from a relative or friend, and getting out into the world a little bit—to get a new haircut, see a movie, visit a museum, take a walk or bike ride—can give you a different perspective on yourself, help you take a realistic look at the shape your body's in. Seeing yourself again as the woman you were before you became a mother may prove very helpful in your efforts to start getting your prepregnancy figure back.

From Your Child's Third Month to Sixth Month

Many child development experts report that at this stage most babies become settled, and you, the new mother, can start living a normal life again. If you are fortunate enough to have a "settled baby" at three months, you are very fortunate indeed, and you probably don't need much extra guidance in sticking to the Post-Pregnancy Diet. If, on the other hand, your baby still seems to be changing routines and schedules almost daily (as my three-month-old certainly did), you may find that much of the advice in the preceding section still applies. Inevitably, you will also discover new changes in your and your baby's lives that will influence your ability to diet.

Many women return to work at some point near when their new babies turn three months old. Most of these women report that returning to work actually helps them diet because they become more active and less homebound. The Post-Pregnancy Diet has special provisions for working mothers who usually eat their mid-day meals away from home, and I think you will find it very easy either to pack your own lunch or order a diet lunch at a restaurant or cafeteria. Here's some additional help with the specifics.

Breast-feeding

If you're returning to work when your baby is three months old, you will probably be cutting down on breast-feeding, or perhaps weaning your baby from the breast entirely. You are likely to feel less hungry as you nurse less, and you can begin to eliminate the supplemental snacks and eat only the three meals plus a New Mom's Milkshake. Stay in touch with your hunger during this phase. Your appetite may wane gradually, rather than abruptly, as your body adjusts to supplying a reduced amount of breast milk or ceases to produce milk. You needn't cut out the supplemental snacks all at once as soon as you start weaning your baby. Eat to meet your appetite, and begin limiting your eating day by day, or week by week, according to your hunger.

If your baby is nursing less or not at all these days, and you are cutting back or eliminating your special snacks, you will, of course, start losing weight more quickly. Sometimes this has the effect of inspiring you to eat less and less so you can lose more and more quickly. It's dangerous to deprive yourself of adequate nutrition at this point, so do stick to the diet and continue to eat to appetite. Remember, nutritionists say it takes up to *eighteen months* for women who have given birth to regain the healthy nutritional status of pre-pregnancy days. Try to eat all the foods specified in the Post-Pregnancy Diet meal plans, and the New Mom's Milkshake. When you feel full and satisfied, stop eating—but don't deny your hunger, which is your body's way of communicating to you that it requires nourishment.

If you are continuing to nurse your baby at this point, without supplementing his/her feedings with formula, he/she is apt to consume more breast milk as he/she gets bigger. Accordingly, your appetite may increase as your body produces more breast milk to meet your growing baby's needs. Stay in touch with your hunger, and use the supplement snacks and milkshakes to help you eat as your appetite dictates. You will continue to lose weight gradually and steadily with this program no matter how long you continue breast-feeding, so try not to become impatient about getting back to your pre-pregnancy weight.

Sometime between four and six months, most pediatricians recommend that babies be introduced to solid foods. As infants begin to take more food in solid form, they usually begin to drink less, so even the nursing baby who is not given formula may start to breast-feed a bit less at some point around six months. When your baby is introduced to juice, nursing may be reduced still more. Be aware of how these changes in your baby's life may change your breast-feeding schedules and frequency, and adjust your eating accordingly. Some babies continue to breast-feed heavily even as they add more and more solid food and juice to their diets, so don't cut back on your supplemental snacks until you perceive a definite change in your baby's nursing needs, and a subsequent change in your own appetite.

Meal Scheduling

If you've returned to work at this point, the workaday routine will impose its own schedule, and your meal times will fall into place: breakfast before you leave in the morning, lunch in the middle of the day, and dinner when you get home in the evening. The Post-Pregnancy Diet is designed so that you can make the transition from mother-at-home to woman-at-work *plus* mother-at-home without skipping a beat in your diet program. You've read in Chapter 2 how to order lunch from a restaurant menu or choose from among cafeteria offerings and how to take your own diet lunch to work with you. If you have business dinners out as well, refer to the Post-Pregnancy Diet guidelines for eating dinner in a restaurant.

If you've gotten into the habit of enjoying your New Mom's Milkshake at mid-morning, or in the afternoon, you can take it to work with you in a thermos, and/or store it in a refrigerator at work. Many new working mothers report that they don't need the snack as much during the day once they're back at work, and they find it an excellent treat to savor as soon as they get home in the evening before preparing supper, or between dinner and bedtime.

Mothers whose maternity leave is longer than three months or who choose to make mothering their full time work may find at this point that meal scheduling takes more time and effort to establish. If your child still sleeps irregularly and feeds on demand, you may still be sleeping and eating at odd hours yourself. Try to stick to the pattern of meal spacing suggested in the previous section by scheduling your meals at four- to five-hour intervals; if you're still having the supplemental snacks, have them at least two hours after the last meal and two hours before the next.

As your baby gets closer to six months, you will probably be starting to schedule his/her meals at times approximating normal meal hours, and you can use this to help yourself get into more consistent meal patterns. Some mothers find they enjoy having their own meals while they feed their young children their cereal and fruit. Other mothers, quite understandably, feel that there's no better appetite suppressant than watching a five-month-old dribble banana down his/her chin.

In any case, as your infant becomes a baby and starts to eat solid food, you can start thinking in terms of family meal times, and your own meal scheduling will probably become more regular. Most new mothers find this helpful in their diet efforts.

Fatigue

Mothers of young children who go back to work full time are bound to be exhausted much of the time. In fact, most of us in this situation find we have two full-time jobs. All too often, you may find yourself very, very tired at the end of a workday—and immediately confronted with a needy baby who's delighted to see you. Since it's usually impossible to take a refreshing nap or rest in the early evening when you often need it most, many new mothers find this a very difficult time to resist snacking. A little bit of food will make you feel better when your energy level is low, so this is an excellent time to enjoy your New Mom's Milkshake. Many new mothers find this the perfect evening "cocktail" that gives them the lift they need to attend to their baby and home in the evening.

All mothers are apt to experience a great deal of fatigue, during the three-to-six-month phase of mothering. Caring for a baby, whether you do it all day long or after working outside the home all day, is truly tiring—and add to this the cumulative effects of having been on an irregular and/or very demanding schedule for several months. The result may be a very tired woman whose diet discipline and motivation are not as strong as she would like them to be.

Again, new mothers *must* focus on getting adequate rest. If you feel you need to go to bed at 8 or 9 P.M., it's better to do that than to try to gain the energy to stay up by nibbling into the evening. On weekends, take naps when the baby does and learn to take ten-minute catnaps whenever you get the chance. Being well rested will help you stay on your diet.

There will probably be a strong temptation to eat to keep yourself awake sometimes—you may feel that a cup of coffee and a piece of cake after dinner will help you enjoy some evening time alone with your husband, for example. But it's important to your dieting efforts to avoid the habit of dealing with fatigue by eating. When you're tired, *sleep*—and try to help your husband, family, and friends understand how important sleep is to your health at this time.

Your Own Time

Now, more than ever, you'll need to take time for yourself. Getting off on your own to enjoy personal time helps you stay in touch with yourself and can increase your body awareness as well as heighten your morale. Make a point of taking some regular time each week to do something you really enjoy; the best is something active that gets you moving around and using your body in new and different ways.

Your everyday schedule may be busier at this point than ever before, and taking time to yourself may seem impossible. But the busier your days and the more obligations you have, the more in need of leisure time to yourself you will be. Many people find that they can't resist overeating when their lives become frantic. If you are one of these people, you must take particular care to find relaxation and your own time regularly. The point is to learn to treat yourself to something other than food, and at this point in new mothering, some extra time to yourself may be the most valuable little gift you can treat yourself to.

From Your Child's Sixth Month to the First Birthday

This is the time, of course, when your baby starts to really change—usually by first sitting up, then crawling, then standing, then taking a few steps. Many mothers find that the rewards of mothering become greater now, and as the baby becomes more active, the demands of taking care of him/her also become greater. Some women who started the Post-Pregnancy Diet soon after their babies were born will find that they have lost most of the weight they needed to lose at this point. Others who started later or had more to lose are bound to find that dieting is becoming quite easy now. Here are some extra tips:

Breast-feeding

If you are breast-feeding now, you will probably continue to have a larger appetite and need the special snacks to keep your hunger satisfied and to insure a good milk supply. Though your baby is larger and drinking more, he or she is probably also eating more solid foods and possibly drinking more juice as well, so you might find that you are becoming gradually less hungry and can begin to cut back on snacks and milkshakes. Be aware of your own appetite as well as your child's changing feeding patterns so you'll be able to determine how much you need to eat these days. And don't feel discouraged if the extra weight doesn't come off as quickly as you'd like. Nursing mothers who aren't on the Post-Pregnancy Diet often don't lose any weight—and may even gain weight!—while they breast-feed their babies.

At this stage of motherhood, some women have weaned their babies to a bottle except for one breast-feeding a day. Many women who are nursing just once a day report that they feel much less hungry than before and don't require any extra snacks or milkshakes. Others find that the three meals a day plus two milkshakes work best for them. Monitor your appetite as your child nurses less and less, and keep track of weekly weight losses. If one week passes and you haven't lost any weight on your own personal formula of diet meals, snacks, and shakes, you are probably eating more than you need and must make an adjustment by eliminating an extra snack or shake.

Meal Scheduling

This is often a time when mothers like to start to get their young children used to the structure of family mealtimes at regular hours of the day. Most children of this age are quite wild when they eat, and their behavior does not lend itself to peaceful mealtimes when you can focus on and enjoy what you are eating. If you are very tolerant, you may not find this a problem, but most new mothers on a diet find it much easier to really savor their diet meals if they eat before or after their young children.

If you choose to have your child eat with you, you'll find that his or her curiosity about what you have on your plate needn't be discouraged, because the Post-Pregnancy Diet has been designed to include wholesome foods that are fine for young children (*if* they have the teeth and eating skills to handle them, of course). But, if you eat with your child, try to keep two rules in mind:

- Stay seated throughout the meal. Constantly getting up to clean up spills on the floor, overturned cups of juice, or whatever, makes chaos of a meal, and prevents you from getting the satisfaction you need from your food.

- *Never* nibble on what your child has left on the plate.

Because children eat so erratically at this age, it can be disturbing to see so much food go to waste, and many new mothers report that they get in the habit of popping stray pieces of carrot or tuna or spaghetti into their mouths, until they find themselves doing it unconsciously. Even if the food your child leaves is part of your meal from the Post-Pregnancy Diet, make a point *not* to eat it.

Several images come to mind when I think of mothers eating their kids' leftovers: I remember picking up pinches of dry Cheerios from the kitchen table where my seven-month-old daughter had spilled them and mindlessly eating them—dry cereal! And I recall watching a mother give her child a bite-size piece of a peanut butter and jelly sandwich at the beach one day. The child looked at the sandwich piece, then dropped it on a towel. Almost as though by instinct, the mother picked it up and ate it herself, then continued eating her own lunch. Children may continue to leave food uneaten for several years to come, and eating it yourself will eventually add many more calories to your diet than you'll want to consume.

One of the purposes of the Post-Pregnancy Diet is to help you become very aware of everything you eat. Be vigilant about not eating food you don't want and probably don't even like, even if your child has left it in front of you.

Fatigue

Children between the ages of six months and a year can require almost constant surveillance. Once they start moving around and discovering one hazard after another, their parents can easily become exhausted just trying to keep an eye on them. This is often a very tiring phase for new moms—but because the child is well out of the infant stage and probably on a fairly regular sleeping and eating schedule, some mothers no longer feel "entitled" to their fatigue.

Just as this diet is designed to help you become increasingly aware of your hunger levels, your experience of motherhood should be helping you to focus more on your need for rest. Again, being tired and having to be awake often sets you up for food temptations that you might not be strong enough to resist. Try not to think about whether you *should* be tired. If you feel the need for rest or sleep, indulge yourself. Adequate rest is essential to your diet efforts, and you'll need to pay attention to your need for it.

Since many children begin to nap less at about this time, you may need to make special provisions to get all the rest you need. Watch for daily patterns in your fatigue. The time when many mothers report feeling most tired is between late afternoon and early evening; interestingly, it's also the time of day when lots of new moms say they are most tempted to go off their diets. If this is true of you, try to make arrangements to get some help at that time of day, so you can give your body what it really needs—rest—rather than subjecting yourself to the temptation to eat something fattening. Paying attention to all your body's needs is an invaluable aid to successful dieting.

Your Own Time

Many new mothers find it gets harder and harder to take time to themselves as their baby's first birthday approaches. Little ones between the ages of six months and a year usually love to be with their mothers and are often utterly uninhibited and irresistible in expressing this desire. Also, because it is a time of "firsts"—first time sitting up, first time standing, then standing and letting go, then taking first steps—you may find yourself spending more and more time with the baby because you don't want to miss anything. Babies of this age have lots of needs, of course, and they can make endless demands. But as much if not more than ever, you need to find times that are reserved for you alone.

So many new mothers say that they find themselves overeating in response to being in a role of constantly giving. It's clear that most moms will need to take small vacations from that role, much as they may enjoy it, if only for the sake of continuing to diet successfully. Becoming reacquainted with the parts of yourself that existed before you were a mother can help you visualize and get back your pre-motherhood body. Enlist help from family and friends, or hire some child care, rather than neglecting your need for time to yourself. It's practically essential to staying on the Post-Pregnancy Diet.

From Your Child's First to Second Year

During this period, your baby starts to become a child, and many mothers find dieting easier. Life is usually somewhat more predictable as daily routines are established, and for the dieting mom, this can mean a greater sense of control that really helps you stick to your diet. Following are some guidelines.

Breast-feeding

When you're nursing a child into the second year, the child is sure to be getting most of his/her nourishment from a variety of solid foods and such liquids as juice and milk. It's very unlikely you'll feel as hungry as you did in the earlier months of breast-feeding. Children's eating patterns may change from month to month, however, and new mothers as well as pediatricians agree that around a child's first birthday, he or she often loses interest in eating solid foods. In some cases, this may mean a temporary increase in nursing, and a mother's concomitant need for more calories. The beauty of this diet is that you can adapt it continuously to your baby's changing nursing needs and your changing appetite.

As before, try to stay aware of your own hunger levels as they correspond to the amount you are nursing. Don't feel discouraged if your appetite keeps changing and, in increasing the amount of snacks and shakes you have, you lose more slowly. Feel good about the fact that you are able to lose weight while you continue to breast-feed, and that you will be that much ahead of the game when you've weaned your baby.

Meal Scheduling

Charming as toddlers are, table manners usually aren't their strong suit, and yet many mothers want to include a child of this age at the family meal. Keep in mind the two rules for having meals with your child in the preceding section of this chapter—stay seated until you've finished eating your meal, and don't touch even a morsel of the food your child disdains.

These days, your meals will probably be scheduled at the usual hours of the day, and with this diet, you will find that your appetite levels quickly become adjusted to a regular schedule of meals. With all the distractions your toddler is apt to come up with at the table, however, do try to focus as much as possible on enjoying your own meal. At this point, the sense of satisfaction of a pleasant mealtime can be almost as important as the physical sensation of being full.

Fatigue

A group of medical researchers once set up an experiment in which professional athletes were instructed to follow toddlers around, imitating their every physical movement. None of the athletes lasted more than a few hours. Every mother of a child aged one to two years can understand why. This is the age of perpetual motion, and just watching your child these days can be exhausting. Unfortunately, physiologists tell us that, tiring though it is, unless you are doing as the athletes did and duplicating every movement, just keeping up with your toddler doesn't really burn very many calories. Although you experience lots of fatigue and frequent feelings of drained energy, you're not really getting the kind of exercise that burns calories. It hardly seems fair.

The best antidote for the kind of fatigue the mother of a toddler is apt to experience is, of course, good rest, and sleep when possible. Your child is probably only taking one nap, or two very brief naps, at this age, and may be staying up a bit later in the evening as well, so you may have to make special arrangements to get all the rest you need.

Whether working outside the home or mothering full time, most new moms find this age very tiring, as well as being lots of fun. Because fatigue can influence your diet motivation and morale, you'll want to find ways to avoid tiredness. The best way is to get the rest you need every day, rather than trying to wait for the weekend to catch up. Your child may still be dictating the early hour that you awaken in the morning, so try to get to bed as early as possible—even if it means giving up some precious evening time to yourself. If you can't get all the sleep you need at night, make a point of taking a nap or lying down for a rest at some point during the day. The best way to avoid letting fatigue overwhelm you is to keep up with it on a day-to-day basis, and this will be a great help to your diet efforts.

Your Own Time

I remember once telling a more experienced mother how hard it was to leave my four-month-old daughter to go into town for a business lunch. "It gets harder as they get older," she warned me, and of course she was right. By the time your child is between the ages of one and two, his physical needs from you may be starting to decrease, but the psychic ties strengthen as the child acquires a real personality and the ability to express love and affection.

At the same time, toddlers are far from being separate and independent individuals, and the demands they make can be truly draining. As before, it is important to your sense of yourself and your own individuality, as well as to your ability to stay in touch with your desire to get back in shape, for you to have some of your own time. At this stage of mothering, trying to do everything can seem to become a way of life, and it may often be hard to choose the best way to use even a few minutes of extra time when you find it. The best weight-loss priorities for a new mom at this point are:

- Keeping your meals as much on schedule as possible

- Resting or sleeping as much as you need to

- Trying to schedule some time to yourself regularly every few days

A full-time mother may only be able to take a ten-minute walk, and a mother who works outside the home may choose to have a cup of coffee or tea after work before heading home. But do make the effort; it can make a big difference in your diet morale.

Your Child's Third Year and Beyond

Do you still qualify as a new mother once your youngest, or only, child is two years old or older? If you're still carrying around weight you gained during your pregnancy, you do. You may be continuing to diet at this point, or you may have just discovered this diet especially designed for new mothers. In either case, you might want some extra pointers on sticking to the diet during this phase of mothering.

Breast-feeding

If you are nursing a child two years old or over, the child is probably getting most of his or her nourishment at meal-times, and breast-feeding probably isn't having a great influence on your appetite. Still, be sure to stay aware of your appetite. If the three meals a day plus one milkshake really leave you feeling hungry, you might need to add an extra shake or a snack until your child is weaned.

Meal Scheduling

By the time your child is two, he or she really is starting to become a little person who participates in family events, including mealtimes. It was at this point that the schedule of our family meals became truly regularized, and I found this most helpful to my dieting efforts.

On weekday mornings, my daughter Polly and I could usually have breakfast together. On weekends, we'd all have breakfast together. I usually ate lunch at my desk at mid-day during the week. (I found it helpful if I stopped working while I ate so I could concentrate on enjoying my food.) At dinner time, I'd sit Polly up on a stool by the kitchen counter and let her eat while I prepared dinner for me and my husband. This meant that Polly and I could socialize while she had dinner, and she could be included in our meal preparations, if not the meal itself—and, best of all, it meant that my husband and I had a civilized dinner on our own later in the evening after Polly had gone to bed.

I think you'll find it really is helpful to your diet if you can adapt a consistent formula to your own household and family schedule. Meal preparations for the Post-Pregnancy Diet never take more than fifteen or twenty minutes, which is about the length of time a young child is willing to spend at a meal, and I know I was much more relaxed at dinnertime when it was just myself and my husband eating together.

I've talked to many mothers who feel differently and like to include their young children at every meal possible, finding it does not necessarily interfere with their ability to be aware of what they're eating and feel satisfied. You can find out what works best for you, of course, by experimenting with different approaches to meal times.

How you schedule your meals while you are on this diet, and afterward when you are maintaining your weight, is bound to help or hinder your ability to take off and keep off extra weight. It's important to figure out what works best for you, and to keep in mind that schedules can always be adapted to suit you and your family's changing needs. But if, by the time your child is two or three years old, you can establish a basic pattern of meals that helps you feel relaxed and content when you are preparing and eating your food, this may help you maintain control over your eating for a long time to come. You may not always be able to adhere to the meal schedule that works best for you, but having a structure to aim for and return to when possible can make ongoing weight control easier than ever.

Fatigue

By the time a child is two, most mothers have found their own ways of successfully dealing with fatigue. Many mothers have perfected the art of ten minute catnaps, or readjusted their evening schedules so that they are always in bed at a time that allows them a good night's sleep.

The best tip I ever got on grabbing some sleep when you need it came from the father of a two-year-old. The advice, for putting yourself to sleep quickly, whether for a long or a short nap, was to lie down, close your eyes, and let your jaw relax so completely that your mouth falls open. Count to twenty mentally, and you're asleep. It really works, and the technique can come in handy especially when you feel "parent's fatigue" but aren't sure you can really get to sleep.

What dieting new mothers should keep in mind about fatigue is that, in addition to being a physical and psychological drain on you, it almost always affects your diet adversely. When you are frequently tired and demoralized, it's almost impossible to control your eating so that you can lose weight, and it's certainly very, very difficult to keep up any kind of regular exercise routine. Again, avoid fatigue by keeping up with your own need for rest. Second only to what you eat, getting enough sleep is an essential element to successful dieting.

Your Own Time

Mothers of children two years old and older have usually figured out how much time they need for themselves and how much time they can really take on a regular basis. What's important is remembering to treat yourself to your own time regularly. When you are a very new mother, many people will advise you to take time to yourself, but as your child gets older, you may need to remind yourself of that advice, balancing it with your many mothering and working responsibilities.

Time to yourself may offer you many pluses that help your diet along, but one essential advantage to taking your own time is that it helps you become more aware of your body. Allowing yourself to experience the dimensions and condition of your body is extremely helpful to getting in shape and staying that way.

Time on your own is important to new mothers and to everyone on a diet. It becomes doubly valuable to dieting new mothers. You can almost always find a way to treat yourself, and it's a small indulgence that really makes the Post-Pregnancy Diet easier. Don't deny yourself as much of your own time as you need and can take.

Chapter 6

~

The Stages-of-Motherhood Guide to Exercise

Everyone who has ever exercised can fully understand the great benefits of being active—your spirits rise, your body feels wonderful, and your energy and stamina are increased. If you're on a diet, losing weight becomes much easier when you include a regular routine of exercise in your diet program. For new mothers who want to lose extra weight gained during pregnancy, the benefits of exercise are practically irresistible. At the same time, most new mothers, and not-so-new mothers as well, find that with everything they have to fit into a single day, there just doesn't seem to be time for exercise.

When I first met Marya Warshaw-Chu and began to attend her classes, my daughter was over two years old and I had reached a plateau in my diet. Attending Marya's postnatal exercise class with women whose babies were only six weeks old, I regretted not having started an exercise program earlier. It seemed to me that new moms who started using their bodies actively as soon as possible after their babies were born could build up strength rather quickly and soon be doing more strenuous (and more calorie-burning) exercise for longer daily sessions.

Marya explained to me that while it is true that we get physically stronger and capable of doing more exercise as our early motherhood progresses out of the postnatal period, our children usually affect our lives in such a way that we have less time to devote to exercise as they get older. It's easy to lay a three-month-old baby on the floor, put on some music, and get involved with a half-hour exercise routine without too many interruptions. A seven-month-old crawler makes this somewhat more difficult, and a year-old toddler can make it virtually impossible.

Because of Marya's extensive pioneering work as a teacher of pre- and postnatal exercise, and because of her own experience as the mother of two, she is highly sensitive to the ways in which a mother's lifestyle may influence her ability to establish a regular daily exercise routine. She realizes that mothers can't always exercise for the same amount of time at the same time every day, and that to admonish them to do so can create the kind of pressure that causes even the most committed exerciser to give up.

Taking all this into account, Marya's general recommendations are as follows:

- Start exercising as soon as you and your physician feel you are ready. Marya's classes start with women four weeks after a vaginal delivery, and six weeks after a cesarean delivery.

- Do only those exercises described here as appropriate to your stage of postnatal readiness; if you have extra time and feel strong enough, you may try extra repetitions of the recommended exercises.

- Move on into succeeding stages of exercise as you feel ready, using the earlier exercises to stretch out and warm up.

- When you have reached the later stages of motherhood, and the entire routine of exercises from beginning to end is appropriate for you, try to find time (about forty-five minutes) at least twice a week when you can do the whole program at one session; your child's naptime may be a good time to do it, or perhaps you can take some time when a babysitter is taking care of your child. On other days, choose three or four favorite exercises that really give you a workout in the areas you most need it and that really feel good to you, and take ten to fifteen minutes to get your body moving with those exercises.

This approach to exercise may not be quite as rigorous as the programs you have been involved with before you had a baby, but it accomplishes the essential goal of getting you moving every day. Once you have begun to get in the habit of including some healthful toning and strengthening movement in your daily schedule, even for fifteen minutes, you will not only look and feel better, you'll also find yourself looking forward to those times when you can devote more time to the full routine.

Marya's philosophy is both realistic and practical. It allows you to proceed at your own pace, and as you will discover, all the exercises—from the very first stretches to the more vigorous exercises designed for later stages—are appropriate for the ways your body has changed after pregnancy.

If your child is six months old or older when you start the Post-Pregnancy Diet and exercise routine, you'll need to start at the beginning along with the moms who are at an earlier postnatal stage. Do as many of these first exercises as you feel comfortable with, adding repetitions and progressing to the succeeding levels as you increase your strength and endurance. Because you are more fully recovered from delivery and birth than the newer moms, you will probably be able to proceed to the later stages and more advanced levels of exercise rather quickly, perhaps moving on to the next level every week or two.

I think most mothers will really enjoy Marya's customdesigned postnatal exercise routine from beginning to end no matter what stage of motherhood they find themselves in when they begin. The exercises here feel great to do and will give you the toning and strengthening benefits you need, in exactly the places you need them.

No exercise program is truly complete without a regular routine of aerobic activity—at best, three forty-five-minute sessions a week, or more. Aerobic exercise increases the output level of your heart and lungs for a sustained period of time, circulating oxygenated blood to your muscles and internal organs, a process that really builds your stamina and helps you overcome fatigue. Aerobic activity also burns calories very efficiently and helps your body keep burning calories even after you've stopped exercising. Best of all for dieters, aerobics have been demonstrated to reduce the appetite, making you feel less hungry and really helping you to cut down on eating. Aerobic activities include walking, cycling, swimming, jogging, running, and calisthenics, to name some of the best.

Your goal will be to have at least three forty-five-minute aerobic workouts each week, but you will want to start slowly and build up gradually. The aerobic activity you select should match your changing levels of strength and endurance at the different stages of motherhood, as well as the changing lifestyle elements that may be involved as your child gets older. For example, with an infant, it may be easiest to take aerobic walks, since you can put the baby in a Gerry pack or Snugli or carriage quite easily. When the child is three to six months old, it might be simplest to use a stationary bike during baby's naptime, or if you are working, in the evening after dinner when the baby is in bed. As your child gets older, it will probably become more convenient to use some of the time when you have a babysitter to get out of the house for a jog, or a swim at a nearby pool. Older toddlers might enjoy doing some parts of an exercise routine with you, especially if there's music, so a video tape of an aerobic dance or exercise class might be best for you at that stage.

As soon as you feel ready to begin aerobic exercise, choose an activity that you'll really enjoy and that seems appropriate to your schedule, and consult with your midwife or doctor for important suggestions on getting started, as well as guidelines for exercising properly at that point in your postpartum period.

Our goal here has been to create an exercise program that offers you all the important toning and strengthening exercises your body needs without overburdening your busy schedule. I think you'll find that the exercises suggested here give you the benefits you need, plus the ease and flexibility that will help you incorporate physical activity into a lifelong program of good health.

If you are a very new mother, check with your doctor. Show her the exercise program in this chapter, then start moving as soon as possible. The special post-pregnancy exercises here will help make your diet easier, more efficient, and a lot more fun!

First Stage-of-Motherhood Exercise Level

If one or two weeks have passed since your vaginal delivery, and you feel ready for some mild abdominal toning exercises as well as some relaxing stretches for the back, and if your doctor or midwife feels you are ready, you will find that these exercises feel great. They're easy, they're relaxing, and they're fun to do. You can even do them in bed if you like.

Tummy Tightener

1. Lie on your back, bending your knees, with feet flat on the floor, lower back resting comfortably against

the floor, and hands resting on the sides of your abdomen.

2. Take a deep breath in through your nose and out through your mouth.

3. Repeat this breath, in through your nose, and as you breathe out through your mouth, tighten your stomach and gently press your waist and lower back into the floor or bed. Relax.

4. Repeat the breath, taking lots of air in through your nose, and as you exhale through your mouth and tighten your stomach, also tighten your vaginal muscles. Relax. (Tightening the vaginal muscles helps you tighten your abdominals in a way you probably can't otherwise.)

Lower Back Lengthener/Abdominal Toner

1. Lie on your back, bending your knees, with feet flat on the floor, lower back resting comfortably against the floor or bed, and arms at your sides.

2. Take a deep breath in through your nose, breathe out through your mouth. As you exhale, tighten your abdominal muscles and press your waist and lower back gently into the floor; press against the floor with your feet, and lift your pelvis up about two inches off the floor, tilted on the diagonal. Hold for one beat, then slowly roll down through the bottom vertebra of your spine. Relax.

3. Repeat the breathing, tilting the pelvis upward, holding the position long enough to relax your shoulders and feel the width of your chest and shoulder blades. Roll down through the bottom vertebra of your spine. Relax.

Abdominal Strengthener

1. Lie on your back, with knees bent, feet flat on the floor or bed, lower back resting comfortably against the floor or bed, and arms at your sides.

2. Breathe deeply and concentrate on relaxing your shoulders and relaxing your neck.

3. Take a deep breath in through your nose, exhale through your mouth, and bring your right knee up to your chest, gently clasping your right knee with both hands and pulling the knee toward you.

4. Let go of your right knee, relax the leg, and return your right foot to the floor in the starting position.

5. Take a deep breath in through your nose, exhale through your mouth, and bring your left knee up to your chest, gently clasping your left knee with both hands and pulling the knee toward you.

6. Let go of your left knee, relax the leg, and return your left foot to the floor in the starting position.

7. Breathe in through your nose, exhale through your mouth, and as you pull your right knee up to your chest and hold it there with your hands, pull your belly in tight and let the back of your waist press into the floor.

8. Holding this position, inhale, then exhale, pulling the belly in, imagining your stomach being very flat, even concave.

9. Release the right knee, relax the leg, and return the right foot to the floor in the starting position.

10. Repeat steps 7, 8, and 9 with the left leg.

11. Next, pull both knees up to your chest, first the right, then the left. Place your hands over your knees and hug them into your chest. Take a big

breath in through your nose, exhale through your mouth, and pull your belly tight and flat into the floor as you pull your knees up a little tighter so that the bottom of your buttocks lift up off the floor.

12. Inhale through your nose, exhale through your mouth, then lift up your head and roll the top of your body up toward your knees as you flatten and tighten your belly. (If your stomach starts to quiver or shake in this position, stop. Relax your body, and return to starting position. It may be too soon for you to do this exercise; just do the first part.)

13. Release both knees, relax legs, and return both feet to the floor in the starting position.

Neck-to-Shoulder Relaxer

1. Sit up, and cross your legs comfortably in front of you, with hands resting on your knees, shoulders down, and head erect and facing front. Slowly and easily, circle your head to the right three times. Circle to the left three times. Breathe easily throughout this exercise.

2. In the same sitting position, take a deep breath through your nose, lift your shoulders up to your ears in a big shrugging movement, and with a big exhalation, let the shoulders drop. Repeat three times.

Second Stage-of-Motherhood Exercise Level

The four gentle exercises just described will be plenty to do in the weeks following your delivery. At about four to six weeks after giving birth, you may feel that you want to do more, and Marya recommends that, at this point, you start concentrating on those exercises you really enjoy doing from among the exercises described here.

In the weeks and months following delivery, she points out, you may have only five minutes a day on certain days that you can spare for exercise. "When women who take my postnatal exercise class ask me what they can do at home, I usually tell them to choose three, four, or five exercises that feel very good to their bodies, that they can remember accurately from class—but also to make sure that one of those exercises is an abdominal exercise. You should feel your abdomen *worked*. That doesn't mean that it should shake, or hurt intensely, but it should feel exercised."

The following series of exercises takes you from the beginning of Marya's postnatal exercise class. This class is designed for women from four weeks after a vaginal delivery, or eight weeks after a cesarean delivery, until six months postpartum.

As you become familiar with the exercises here, you'll notice which feel best to you and make you feel best. You'll want to choose three or four of these exercises to use as a daily core program for yourself, one you can run through on those days when you have only five or ten minutes for exercise. On days when you have more time, you'll want to do the whole series and feel your body start to regain strength and flexibility.

The Big Stretch

1. Stand with your feet hip-width apart, arms relaxed by your sides. Take a deep breath in and lift your arms from your sides upward toward the ceiling. Exhaling deeply, bring the outstretched arms down to the front of your body; with hands flexed upward, push and press at the air in front of you in a continual motion. Bend your knees and drop your

head between your arms. Pull your belly in toward your belly button and up toward your ribs; relax your shoulders. As you complete the exhalation, return to starting position, arms at your sides.

2. Breathe in deeply, lift your arms up, and reach toward the ceiling; exhale, and push the air away with the heels of your hands. Then bend your knees, drop your head, and lift your belly in tightly. As you complete the exhalation, return to starting position, arms at your sides.

3. Take a deep breath, lift your arms up toward the ceiling, and, exhaling, reach toward the ceiling with each arm, stretching up through your fingertips, alternating right and left arm reaches eight times. Complete the exhalation and return to starting position.

4. Breathe in deeply and lift both arms up toward the ceiling; exhale and bring your arms down in front of you, dropping your head between them. Bend your knees slightly and roll your body down slowly, unfolding the vertebra of your back until your upper body is hanging downward, loose and relaxed through the back, neck, shoulders, head, and arms. Breathe in, exhale, and pull your belly in tight as you begin to slowly curl upward, lifting your upper body toward the upright position, knees still bent until you are standing up, arms at your sides.

5. Repeat steps 3 and 4, twice more.

Shoulder Relaxer

1. Stand with your feet hip-width apart, arms relaxed by your sides; inhale and lift your shoulders up to your ears; exhale and release your shoulders. Repeat four times.

2. In the same position, circle your shoulders backward, lifting them up and to the front, then circling them to the back. Repeat eight times, breathing in and out with each circling motion.

3. Place your hands on your shoulders and circle the elbows from the back to the front, lifting the elbows and slowly circling them forward. Repeat eight times, breathing in and out with each circling motion.

4. Stand in the starting position, arms relaxed at your sides; breathe in, and as you exhale, turn your head to the right so that you are looking over your right shoulder, then return to facing front. Breathe in, and as you exhale, turn your head to the left so that you are looking over your left shoulder, then return to facing front. Repeat once more to the right, once more to the left.

5. Breathe in, exhale, and tilt your head back as far as possible, looking up at the ceiling, shoulders relaxed. Breathe in again, and as you exhale, bring your head forward to let it drop in front of you, shoulders relaxed, so that you are looking at the floor. Repeat once more back, once more forward.

Neck-to-Waist Stretcher

1. Stand with your feet hip-width apart, arms relaxed by your sides, head facing forward. Breathe in, and exhale as you bend your right ear to your right shoulder, keeping your left shoulder down to feel the stretch in your neck. Reach your right arm over your head so that your hand rests on your left ear; gently pull your head to the right. Breathe in, and as you exhale, pull your belly button back toward your waist, lifting your belly and bending your knees, as you reach your left arm out to the left, hand flexed upward. Breathe in, and as you exhale, stretch

your left arm upward, slowly arching to the right. Let your right arm drop down to your side, and start to round your back over your legs, dropping both arms, then dropping your head and shoulders, so that your upper body hangs down toward the floor with knees bent. Breathe in, exhale, and roll up slowly, knees bent, until you are standing upright in the starting position, arms relaxed at your sides, head facing front.

2. Repeat this exercise, starting on the left side, beginning by bending the left ear to the left shoulder. Repeat twice on each side.

Pelvis Tilt

1. Stand with your feet hip-width apart, hands on your hips. Bend your knees slightly, breathe in, and as you exhale, tilt your pelvis forward, tightening your belly. Release your pelvis, knees still bent. Breathe in, exhale, and tilt your pelvis upward, flattening your abdomen, pulling your belly button in toward your back.

2. Repeat four times.

Pelvis Switch

1. Stand with your feet hip-width apart, hands on your hips. Bend your knees slightly, breathe in, and as you exhale, move your right hip to the right and slightly upward, then back to center. Breathe in, exhale, and move your left hip to the left and slightly upward, then back to center.

2. Repeat four times.

Hip Circles

1. Stand with your feet hip-width apart, hands on your hips. Bend your knees slightly, breathe in, and as you exhale, circle your hips around to the right four times, moving to the right, to the rear, and to the left. As you circle forward, tighten the muscles just under your buttocks.

2. Return to starting position; bend your knees slightly, breathe in, and as you exhale, circle your hips to the left four times, moving to the left, to the rear, and to the right. As you circle forward, tighten the muscles just under the buttocks.

Shake Out

1. Your lower back should be feeling nice and relaxed at this point, and it's a good time to shake out all your body.

2. Shake your legs one at a time by lifting them up off the ground and just shaking.

3. Shake out your hands by letting them flop back and forth at the wrists.

4. Shake your arms out, and shake your shoulders up and down and in every direction.

5. Let your jaw drop and shake your head and face out.

6. Keep all your muscles loose as you shake out all of your body. It should feel really good—and it's fun! (Your baby will really love watching you shake out all over!)

Toe Taps

1. Stand with your feet directly under your pelvis, just a few inches apart, arms relaxed by your side. Lift

and tighten your belly, keep your spine long, and relax your shoulders. Breathe in and out evenly as you stretch your right foot forward, pointing your toes on the floor, heel off the ground. Keep the weight centered in your hips as you point your toes, then flex your foot. Point and flex eight times, ending with the foot pointed. Lift the pointed toes up a few inches and tap them down onto the floor eight times; return your leg to the starting position.

2. Repeat the exercise by pointing and flexing your left foot eight times, tapping your toes eight times. Return your leg to the starting position.

Knee Lifts

1. Stand with your feet directly under your pelvis, just a few inches apart, arms relaxed by your side. Lift and tighten your belly, keep your spine long, and relax your shoulders. Breathe in and out evenly as you lift your right knee straight up, as though there were a string attached to your knee and pulling it upward; then set it down. Repeat lifting and lowering eight times.

2. Repeat the exercise with your left knee, lifting and lowering eight times.

3. Shake your right leg out loose, then shake your left leg out loose.

Knee Bends

1. Stand with your feet spread wider than your hips, toes pointed slightly outward, belly lifted and held in, and arms extended to the sides. Breathe in and out evenly as you shift your weight to the right, bending your right knee over your right foot, keeping your left leg straight. Shift to the left, bending

your left knee over your left foot. Then return to center and bend both knees over both feet; then straighten up, and repeat—to the right, the left, and center, feeling the heel of the straight leg press down into the floor to work the inner leg—eight times.

2. Repeat the exercise, shifting from right to left, bending your right knee over your right foot, your left knee over your left foot, alternating sides without bending both knees over both feet in the center. Shift from right to left, then left to right eight times. Return to the starting position.

3. Bend forward, keeping a flat back, arms extended to the sides, belly lifted, and continue alternating knee bends to the right and left, eight times.

4. Now, as you alternate bending your knees from right to left, swing your arms in a windmill fashion so that you reach for the bent knee with the opposite hand. As you bend your right knee over your right foot, back flat, belly lifted, reach for your right knee with your left hand, stretching your right hand up and back behind you, turning your head to look at the hand behind you. As you bend your left knee over your left foot, back flat, belly lifted, reach for your left knee with your right hand, stretching your left hand up and back behind you, turning your head to look at the hand behind you. Repeat eight times.

5. Return to the starting position: feet spread wider than hips, toes pointed slightly outward, belly lifted and held in, arms extended to the sides. Bend both knees over both feet, and breathe evenly as you lift the heels up off the floor and lower them down again, eight times. Repeat eight bended knee heel lifts in sets of eight, four times.

6. Shake your right leg loose, then your left leg.

Two-Minute Free Movement

At this point in the postnatal class, Marya does a free movement phase. This is how she describes it:

"You can do the free-movement phase at home by turning on some music that you enjoy. You can use skips, you can use little bounces, you can walk, you can swing your baby in the air. The point is to try to keep yourself moving for two minutes. Set a timer, or keep an eye on a digital clock. The point isn't to build aerobic endurance, but rather to feel a flow and a grace and a comfort through your whole body, to enjoy your body through motion. Change from place to place in the room. Try some swings in the body. Try letting your arms swing back and forth, and your hips sway back and forth, and your waist twist. Try lifting the leg up and putting it down; try dropping down to the floor and rolling back up. As you move, feel your belly very lifted and flat, while the rest of your body feels very free in the space. Have fun with this movement, but *keep moving* until the two minutes are up."

Following the free movement, shake your body out—each of your legs, each of your arms, your shoulders, your head, your hands and feet.

Calf Stretches

1. From a standing position, extend your left foot forward, foot flat on the floor, toes pointing forward, so that your left foot is about two to three feet in front of your right foot. Keep your right foot flat on the floor, toes pointing forward, and bring your weight forward over your left knee, keeping your right leg straight. Place your hands on your left thigh and feel the stretch in the right calf. Breathe evenly as you gently stretch the calf.

2. Repeat the exercise on the other side, extending the right foot forward to stretch the left calf.

Sitting Position Warm-Up

1. Sit on the floor with your legs crossed, your spine very straight, hands resting easily on your knees, belly lifted. Raise your shoulders up to your ears, and release them; repeat lifting and releasing the shoulders. Let your chin fall to your chest, and feel the stretch in the back of your neck.

2. Lift your head up and bend your right ear to your right shoulder. Bring your head to the center, and bend your left ear to the left shoulder, then return to starting position, head upright, facing forward.

Pelvic Roll

1. Sit on the floor with your legs crossed, your spine very straight, hands resting easily on your knees, belly lifted. Breathe in, exhale, and round your back, dropping your head and tightening your belly so that the abdominal muscles are helping you hold the position. Don't hold onto your knees with your hands; keep your hands relaxed so your stomach muscles do the work. Breathe in, and as you exhale, roll back up to a straight spine. Repeat rounding your back, dropping your head to roll your pelvis back, and tightening your abdominals three more times. On the fourth roll back, hold the position.

2. In the rolled-back position, weight on your buttocks, shoulders relaxed, hands resting on your knees, take a deep breath, exhale, and tighten the vaginal muscles. Holding these muscles tight, try to tighten the muscles that are underneath your belly button. Holding these muscles tight, take a deep breath, exhale, and roll up to a straight spine. Release the muscles, breathe in, exhale, roll down, and tighten the vaginal and center-abdominal muscles again; holding the muscles tight, roll up to a straight spine and release. Repeat the exercise a total of four times.

Waist Stretch

1. Sitting on the floor with your legs crossed, your spine very straight, arms at your sides, hands flat on the floor, belly lifted, breathe in deeply; exhale and reach across with your right arm to place your right hand on the floor near your left knee. Bend your left elbow slightly, and reach out through your right fingertips, stretching from the bottom of your right hip and the right side of your waist, keeping your belly lifted. Hold the stretch to a count of eight, feeling the muscles engaged, but not hurting; if you feel pain, ease back a bit. Return to starting position.

2. Repeat the exercise, reaching across with your left arm, holding for a count of eight. Return to starting position.

3. Take a deep breath in, exhale, lift and tighten the belly, and roll down so that your forehead reaches for your left knee, hands resting on the floor, shoulders relaxed, stretching from the bottom of the spine; roll up to a straight spine. Repeat, rounding over toward your right knee, and roll up to a straight spine.

4. Uncross your legs and shake them out loose.

Foot Flexes

1. Sit on the floor with your legs stretched out straight in front of you, keeping your back very straight and your belly lifted. Bend your right knee into your body and take hold of it with both hands, pulling it in, right foot flat on the floor, with your left leg stretched straight out in front, lifted off the floor about an inch, toes pointed. Circle your left foot around easily, using your toes to draw a circle in a

clockwise direction; circle eight times. Reverse, circling eight times in a counterclockwise direction. Flex your left toes so they are spread and pointing upward, stretching back toward you; now point your toes. Alternate flexing and pointing eight times. Lower your leg, shake it out.

2. Pull your left knee toward your body, holding it with both hands. Pull it in, left foot flat on the floor, with the right leg stretched straight out in front, lifted off the floor about an inch, toes pointed. Repeat the above exercise with the right leg. Lower the leg and shake it out.

Belly Tightener

1. Sit on the floor with your legs stretched out straight in front of you, back very straight, and belly lifted. Bring the bottoms of the feet together so you are sitting in a tailor position, knees bent out to the sides. Place the palms of your hands together at chest level, elbows bent and lifted. Take a deep breath in, exhale, and press the palms of your hands together, letting your belly curve backward away from your hands, and rounding your back. Hold the position, breathing evenly, for a count of eight. Roll up to a straight spine, and roll back again, holding for eight counts. (If your belly begins to shake too much, come out of this position right away; roll up and shake your hands out loose, and relax your belly.)

2. Roll down as described above, belly curved in, spine rounded, palms of your hands pressed together; hold the position, and stretch your arms straight out in front of you, making fists with your hands. Then take your right foot and place it on the floor with your right knee bent; place your left knee on the

floor with the left knee bent, so that your fists are held next to your bent legs just outside the knees. Roll your back down a little farther, spine rounded, belly lifted and tight. Take a deep breath in, exhale, and move your fists up and down, pressing the air, keeping your arms parallel with the floor, blowing out through your mouth each time you push your fists down. Press your fists up and down eight times, and eventually, try to work up to sixteen times. (If this hurts your lower back, or your belly shakes too much, come out of the position immediately.) Roll up, stretch your legs out, and gently round your body forward over the legs, relaxing all your muscles, breathing easily.

Spine Expander

1. Sit on the floor with your legs spread as wide apart as you can comfortably stretch, back very straight, belly lifted. Breathe in deeply, exhale, and round your head down toward your right knee, feeling the stretch in your back. Reach out with your left hand for the inside of your right ankle, keeping your right hand flat on the floor, just outside your right knee. Keep your head dropped down, neck relaxed. Press your left hip gently against the floor to feel the stretch; keep your belly lifted. Take thirty-two long, steady stretches out toward your right foot, breathing evenly, (don't bounce!) and slowly lift up to starting position.

2. Repeat the exercise on the other side, reaching out with your right hand for the inside of your left ankle. Return gently to starting position.

3. Round forward, letting your head drop down toward the floor between your legs, your arms relaxed, hands resting on either leg. Slowly roll up, close the legs, and shake them out loose.

Third Stage-of-Motherhood Exercise Level

The following series of exercises is designed for women who have given birth at least six months ago. If your youngest or only child is six months or older when you begin the Post-Pregnancy Diet and Exercise Program, and you have not exercised since your last delivery, it is suggested that you do the First and Second Stage exercises for a few weeks before starting the Third Stage series. If you have been doing some exercise since the birth of your last child, you may begin with the exercises here. The exercise routine incorporating all three stages, from first to third, creates a complete series that takes about forty-five minutes and makes an excellent total routine you'll want to do in its entirety when time permits.

If you have been doing the Second Stage-of-Motherhood Exercise series for the past six months, you have probably chosen your favorite three or four exercises that you try to do daily. This third-level series will add more exercises to your repertoire so that you can try some new favorites for your short daily workout.

Before you start the Third Stage-of-Motherhood Exercises, you should repeat three exercises from the First Stage-of-Motherhood Exercise Level series. Go back to the beginning of this chapter and do one exercise from each of the following three categories:

• Tummy Tightener

• Lower Back Lengthener/Abdominal Toner

• Abdominal Strengthener

These exercises will help you stretch out your lower back and rework your abdominal muscles in preparation for the following, more demanding exercises.

Thigh Tightener

1. Lie on your back, bend your knees, feet flat on the floor, lower back resting comfortably against the floor, arms at your sides. Bring both knees up to your chest, then stretch both legs up toward the ceiling with feet flexed. Breathing evenly, alternate pointing and flexing the feet eight times, keeping the abdomen pulled in, lower back pressed into the floor.

2. On the eighth foot flex, hold the position, and open your legs about one foot apart. Bring your flexed feet together using the inner thigh muscles to pull the legs in. Repeat opening and closing eight times, breathing evenly, feeling your belly tight and flat, your lower back pressed into the floor. Lower the legs, knees bent, feet flat on the floor.

Pelvis Bridge

1. Lie on your back, knees bent, feet flat on the floor, lower back resting comfortably against the floor, arms at your sides. Breathe in deeply and exhale. Pull in the belly and tilt the pelvis upward as far as you can without lifting the back of the waist from the floor. Feel the stretch in the backs of your thighs down into your buttocks. Now let your buttocks drop about two inches, and lift your pelvis up again; drop it, and repeat lifts eight times, exhaling with each lift.

2. On the eighth lift, hold the position, breathe in deeply, exhale, and press the knees together, feeling the inner muscles of your thighs tighten to bring the legs together. Open again, then close a total of eight times, exhaling each time you bring the knees together.

3. After closing the eighth time, open your knees, breath in deeply, exhale, and gently push your pelvis upward another inch. Then slowly roll your back down, vertebra by vertebra, to the starting position. Shake out your legs, relaxing your back and abdomen.

Back Relaxer

1. Lie on your back, knees bent, feet flat on the floor, lower back resting comfortably against the floor; stretch your arms out so they are opened to the side. Breathing evenly, turn your head to look at your left hand, and let both knees fall to the right. Hold for a few seconds, then bring the head and knees to the starting position in the center.

2. Turn your head to look at your right hand. Let both knees fall to your left, hold, and roll back to center. Repeat four times on each side.

Buttocks Toner

1. Lie on your right side, propping up your upper body on your right elbow, your left hand flat on the floor in front of your chest, legs together, knees bent up, belly lifted. Straighten your left leg, the one on top, stretching it down directly from your hip. Flex your left foot, and keeping the leg parallel to the floor, knee facing forward, raise and lower the leg one inch up, one inch down, sixteen times.

2. Keeping your left leg straight and stretched out, point your toe, keep the leg parallel to the floor, knee facing forward, and raise and lower the leg one inch up, one inch down, sixteen times. Hold the leg in this position.

3. Keeping your left leg straight and stretched out, toe pointed, make sixteen circles in one direction with

the toe, then sixteen circles in the opposite direction. Bend your knee back in, rub the left buttock and hip to relieve the tension, and relax your body.

4. Repeat steps 1, 2, and 3 lying on your left side, working the right leg.

Buttocks Stretcher

1. Lie on your right side, propping up your upper body on your right elbow, your left hand flat on the floor in front of your chest, legs together, knees bent up, belly lifted. Straighten your left leg, the one on top, stretching it down directly from your hip, foot flexed. Rotate the leg so that the knee is facing upward, the toes are facing upward, the leg is turned upward from hip to foot. Bend your knee, bringing it in toward the shoulder, and grasp your leg under the knee with the right hand. Gently pull the knee in, breathing evenly, to stretch the underneath part of your buttock. Relax the leg in toward your shoulder, and release.

2. Repeat this stretch, lying on your left side, stretching your right buttock.

Outer Thigh Toner

1. Lie on your right side, propping up your upper body on your right elbow, your left hand flat on the floor in front of your chest, legs together, knees bent up, belly lifted. Straighten your left leg, the one on top, stretching it down directly from your hip, foot flexed, then swing the leg forward to the front so that it's at a right angle to your body. Lift and lower the leg sixteen times, breathing evenly, belly pulled in. Point your foot, and lift and lower sixteen times, breathing evenly, belly pulled in. Cir-

cle the pointed toe sixteen times in one direction, then sixteen times in the opposite direction. Bend your knee in, relax.

2. Repeat the exercise lying on your left side, working the right leg.

Upper Thigh Workout

1. From lying flat on the floor face down, come up into the hydrant position on all fours with your weight on your hands and knees, belly lifted, back flat, head held level with the shoulders. Lift your right knee so that the upper thigh is parallel to the floor, knee bent upward, foot flexed. Breathing evenly, lift your leg up about two inches, keeping your belly tightened and lifted. Lower the leg two inches, lift and lower, sixteen times. Place your knee down on the floor.

2. Repeat the exercise lifting your left knee.

3. From the hydrant position, shift your weight all the way back toward your feet so that your buttocks are resting on your heels, hands still flat on the floor in front of you, head dropped down between the outstretched arms. Breathe evenly as you focus on your lower back, holding the position as you breathe to a count of sixteen.

Back-of-the-Legs Toner

1. From the hydrant position, on your hands and knees—belly lifted, back flat, head level with your shoulders—curl your toes under. Shift your weight back onto your feet, raising your buttocks, hands still flat on the floor in front of your, head and neck relaxed between the arms. Your heels will come up

off the floor as you assume this position; breathing evenly, belly lifted, alternate pressing first your right heel, then your left heel, into the floor, alternating sixteen times.

2. Press both heels down, and walk your hands back to your feet. Drop your head down, shoulders, neck, and arms relaxed, loose as a rag doll, holding some tension in the legs to keep them straight. Breathe evenly in this very relaxed position to a count of eight. Bend the knees and roll up slowly through the spine, keeping the belly lifted.

3. When you are standing upright, shake everything loose: Pick up each leg and shake it; shake your arms, your face, your shoulders. Take a big stretching yawn, lifting up your arms, yawn through your mouth and through your body. Relax.

This is the end of the exercise routine. Once you are familiar with how to do them, it will probably take you about forty-five minutes to do all the exercises from beginning to end. When you do all the exercises together consecutively, try to keep up a rhythm without taking breaks between individual exercises or series. The routine is paced to relax certain parts of the body that have been worked out, while still keeping you moving. You'll find that it feels terrific to do it from beginning to end.

Remember, once you're experienced with these exercises, even at the very first level, select a few—three or four—that you really like, and that you really will do every day when you have a few minutes to spare. (Ten minutes is all you really need to do a series of three or four exercises, and even the busiest mom can find ten minutes a day.) Your schedule and your free time will vary from day to day; that's the one thing you can count on, so you'll want to be very familiar with a few exercises you can do anytime, whenever you can fit them in.

Otherwise, try to make time for yourself—either baby's regular naptime, or babysitter time—twice a week for forty-five minutes to do the whole routine. Also, keep in mind that as your baby gets older, she will be fascinated with what you're doing, especially if you turn on some lively music. At the toddler stage, children love to imitate and will often join right in, which can really make your exercise period fun.

When you select the exercises that you will try to do every day, choose exercises that work out various parts of your body: one exercise for your belly, one that stretches out your spine, one for your legs, one for your buttocks. Make yourself feel good by establishing the exercises you will do on a daily basis—they can change from week to week, if you like—and saying to yourself, "I will do these four exercises every day without fail!" Stick to it, have fun with it, and see what a difference it can make in your feelings about your diet and your body.

Video Recommendations

It's not all that easy to find a videotape of aerobic exercise that's really best for you. The smart approach, of course, is to rent a variety of exercise videos that look interesting, try the routines, and find one that works for you.

Marya offers some general guidelines in choosing a safe and effective exercise tape: Always look for an aerobic routine that is "low-impact." What that means is that you are not stressing joints and muscles by pounding your body against the hard surface of the floor (particularly unsafe for women who have recently given birth because hormonal levels influence joint and muscle strength and may make these parts of the body more vulnerable than usual). The way to be sure an exercise program is low-impact is to watch the exercises and make sure that one foot is always on the floor; at no time, should both feet be lifted from the floor at the same time.

Adequate stretching and warming up is another element to look for in a routine. About one-sixth to one-quarter of the length of the entire routine should be spent stretching and warming up. If the routine is an hour long, the stretch/warm-up should be a minimum of 10 to 15 minutes long; for a half hour workout, at least 5 to 8 minutes of stretching and warming up should be offered.

Finally, make sure the exercises you're doing don't cause severe or sharp pains while you're doing them, especially in the lower back; there, you shouldn't feel any pain or pulling sensations at all. If an exercise does hurt your back, stop doing it immediately and skip that particular movement the next time you do that routine. If several of the exercises hurt or pull your back, you should look for a new routine. Responsible instructors usually make sure none of their exercises will hurt or injure your back, but some people have more back strength than others, so you have to be your own judge.

Following is a list of some of the videos I've found helpful for my home workouts. Some of them included a few exercises that were too hard on my back, and some of them showed high-impact movements that I simply skipped. To keep up aerobic benefits while the video instructor demonstrated an exercise I didn't want to do, I'd just repeat an exercise demonstrated earlier to keep myself moving.

Start Up with Jane Fonda,
Lorimar Home Video, Lightyear Entertainment

This is my favorite of the Fonda videotapes for several reasons. The length—twenty-five minutes—is perfect for new mothers, and combined with alternate-day aerobic routines (like stationary bicycling, jogging, swimming), this routine provides important body benefits. There is a focus on toning arms, legs, hips, buttocks, and stomach, which will be appreciated by new mothers, and, the program emphasizes the benefits of flexibility, balance, and posture. Jane Fonda takes a responsible attitude toward exercise and all her routines are based on the low-impact principle. There is sufficient warm-up, and the pace is just right for women starting to get themselves back in shape. Some exercises may be stressful to some women's backs; stop if you feel any pulling or pain in your back. *Jane Fonda's Pregnancy, Birth and Recovery Workout* tape is, of course, an obvious choice for new mothers, and is also a good routine, but for newcomers to exercise, the *Start Up* tape is the one I recommend.

Kathy Smith's Tone Up, Video Learning Systems, Inc.

This exercise video begins with a good introductory section on keeping your workout safe and not over-stressing your body. The only equipment you need, in addition to proper clothing and aerobic shoes, are some heavy-duty rubber bands for resistance exercise and a pair of weight-lifting or other gloves to protect your hands when you use the rubber bands in some (optional) sections of the program. The warm-up moves pretty quickly, and you might find it takes time to master some of the movements, but the exercises are likely to stay challenging for a long time, and that can help stave off boredom. Three different aerobics classes are featured on the tape; each starts with a few simple movements to which more involved movements are added with repetitions of the initial routines. Lots of popular dance-like movements and rousing music help keep enthusiasm up. Detailed instructions are offered frequently during repetitions to help you check your form. Called "Body Checks," they give you the feeling of personalized attention from an exercise instructor. Ms. Smith also demonstrates how to take and evaluate your pulse at various intervals in the exercise routines. The group of four very in-shape participants led by Kathy Smith creates an atmosphere of being in a class. The exercise routine for stomachs and legs/ buttocks will be of particular interest to lots of new mothers.

The Firm Aerobic Workout with Weights, Meridian Films, Inc.

Weightlifting workouts have the advantage of keeping you physically challenged. As your body becomes stronger and you find the exercises too easy, you can change to heavier weights. This videotape is very handsome and offers clear instructions and a class-like atmosphere. About twenty people are shown in a class led by instructor Susan Harris. Beginners don't use weights for the first week, then begin to gradually add weights to the various exercises. There are good warm-up and cool-down periods, pulse checks are given at several intervals, and the floor exercises are excellent for toning and strengthening. Some of the jumping movements in the early part of the aerobic section are not low-impact, but you can substitute the previous jog-in-place exercise during these jumps. The equipment you need includes a 24-inch board of 2-inch by 4-inch measurements as a shoulder and heel rest, plus the various weights. A forty-minute explanation session at the end of the tape explains which weights to start with, as well as offering lots of useful explanations about weight use, exercise in general, and which exercises work which muscles.

Aerobicise, The Beginning Workout,
Paramount Home Video

This video offers two different classes, the first with four women demonstrating the exercises, and the second with a couple doing the exercises together. Dissolves and interesting camera angles make this tape interesting to watch and prevents the boredom of watching people facing you doing movement repetitions, but inexperienced exercisers may find it confusing and hard to follow, especially in segments in which there are no spoken instructions or counting. A section on sit-ups at the end of the aerobics section of the first class gives excellent instructions for this tummy tightener and demonstrates a multitude of variations on the abdominal exercise, with counting and music to make it easier. New mothers are apt to find this particularly helpful. I doubt that many new mothers can arrange their schedules to provide for time when they can exercise with their husbands, but this tape is certainly for those who can. And, for those who can't, it's pleasant to watch a couple exercising together; the movements can also be done solo.

Videocycle: Competition 1, and *Videocycle: Hawaii, The Big Island,* Cycle Vision Tours, Inc.

These two 60-minute tapes really add interest to cycling on a stationary bike. Experts say that you get the best training effects and aerobic benefits when you really focus on the exercise you're doing while you do it. These tapes offer this advantage over watching TV programs or reading a magazine while you pedal. They really help you focus on your body and your movements, and they help prevent boredom by offering interesting environments. "Competition 1" definitely puts you in an exciting cycle race, and "Hawaii" takes you on a tour of a very

beautiful place. Instructions on good cycling form, pleasant music, a varied terrain including uphill situations
(during which you can increase the tension of your fly-
wheel) and downhill coasting (at lowered tension) all
contribute to holding your interest. Instructions for taking your pulse and on-screen pulse checks at various
intervals in your cycling help you keep track of your
fitness level. The "Hawaii" tape also offers a chart that
targets heart rates for age as well as suggesting six good
stretching exercises to warm up before you begin stationary cycling.

Chapter 7

⌒

Your New,
New Mother's Figure

You can remain on the Post-Pregnancy Diet for as long as it takes for you to get into the shape you want. But almost every dieter worries that once the unwanted weight is lost and the diet is over she will regain all those pounds. On many diets, this is a real concern, but on this special diet for new mothers, you will find that both your tastes and your habits have changed for the better after even a very short time on this weight-loss program.

You will find that your appetite has become geared to a three-meals-a-day schedule and that you no longer think about food between meals. Your taste for sweet and/or fatty foods diminishes greatly, and usually disappears eventually. Eating in a healthful way that keeps you at your desired weight will be easier than ever.

There are really only a few things you need to remember to stay on a good weight-maintenance program when you have completed the diet. First, you will want to restrict your intake of fats and sugary foods. These foods become quite unappealing to dieters after a period of abstinence, so they won't be hard to resist. There may be times when you want a bite of this or that, but try to limit yourself to just a small amount of foods high in fat and/or sugar. You'll probably find that they no longer taste very good to you.

It's important to keep in mind that enjoying your food

helps to make you feel more satisfied. If you can concentrate on what you are eating, really take the time to savor the taste and texture of your food, you'll discover that the food is much more satisfying than when you rush through a meal without thinking about it. To help yourself enjoy everything you eat, focus on eating slowly, and try to arrange an environment that is pleasant and calm for your meals.

Once you have lost the weight you intended to lose you will have proven to yourself that you really can take control over your eating behavior. And, this accomplishment should give you the confidence to know that you can continue to maintain control over your eating and your weight. Sticking to this diet and losing the extra pounds you gained during pregnancy shows how very competent you are at dieting. Your improved appearance and health will be constant reminders of your ongoing success in maintaining your figure.

Arriving at a weight that's healthy and attractive for you personally is the ultimate reward of the Post-Pregnancy Diet. The wonderful feeling of getting your figure back, combined with the emotional high that accompanies your success at dieting, should make you feel terrific about yourself. Sticking to a diet, even a diet that's as easy and pleasant as this one, isn't easy in the midst of a new mother's busy life. It's taken patience and commitment to get your shape back to where you want it, and you should congratulate yourself for this achievement. And while successful dieters can never rest on their laurels entirely, Post-Pregnancy Dieters can certainly relax about their weight when they've completed their diet.

The reason is simple. This diet has reeducated you in the kind of food choices you make, the way you prepare these foods, and your attitude toward eating. Just by following this diet, you've already broken most of the bad habits that probably contributed to your overgain during pregnancy. At this point, you've already developed a taste for wholesome, low-calorie foods. You've learned how to prepare them so that they taste delicious to you and your family. And you now know that you can lose weight without feeling hungry all the time. All the important groundwork for maintaining your weight has been done for you.

This is not the kind of diet that ends with you feeling uncontrollable impulses to rush out and binge on all the foods you were denied while you were losing weight. Your tastes in food as well as your attitude toward food have changed while you were dieting, and these temptations have greatly diminished. Also, because you have been losing weight gradually and consistently, you needn't fear the kind of rapid re-gains that often occur with quick-weight-loss diets. You won't start gaining as soon as you start eating "normally" again. You'll find that your normal eating patterns now really do conform to the basic principles of the diet.

Nonetheless, maintaining your weight will take some thought and effort. You shouldn't find maintenance difficult, but it might be helpful to keep a few tips in mind. Here are some suggestions you might want to refer to from time to time:

- In general, think of your weight maintenance period as a lifelong program of healthful diet and exercise. The best maintenance rules to follow are those of the special "weekends off" featured in the Post-Pregnancy Diet. All you have to remember are the few simple guidelines: no fats, no sugars, no snacking. If you need some ideas or inspiration, refer to Chapter 4, "Weekend Strategies and Forbidden Foods."

- Keep your kitchen stocked with the healthful foods you can enjoy at mealtimes, plus your favorite ingredients for preparing them. Enlist family members to help in keeping fattening foods out of the house. Or, have them all stored in a specific place that's out of sight.

- During times such as on holidays when there are lots of food temptations and at least one large meal to get through, it may be helpful to go back on the formal diet for several days before and after the big festivities. This will help you lose a few of the pounds you might have gained, and just as important, it will diminish your interest in the high-fat and sugary foods that tend to be plentiful during holiday celebrations.

- Similarly, when you know you're facing a big dinner out, have a Post-Pregnancy Diet breakfast and lunch that day and the following day. Going on a "mini-diet" before and after times when you are apt to be faced with lots of food can help you maintain your weight.

- Whenever you can, make family activities and celebrations centered on diversions that don't involve food. As your child gets older, you will find that there are lots of things to do together that offer good exercise and aren't related to eating. Walking, biking, skating, sledding, dancing, and just playing in a park all keep you moving and needn't involve snacking.

The Post-Pregnancy Diet made all your food choices for you and offered you set meal plans to follow during the week, then gave you the freedom to choose your own foods and combinations and your own schedule for eating on weekends. As you conclude the diet and get ready for a lifetime of weight maintenance, you will appreciate more than ever the good training you received on your weekends off. You *know* how to follow healthful, slimming guidelines and stick to a good eating program without following specific meal plans every day—because you've already done it every weekend of your diet! You know you can manage your eating without the imposed structure of a formal diet. More than ever before, you're prepared to keep your weight down through a healthy, wholesome, and sensible eating program.

You'll have plenty of motivation for keeping your new, Post-Pregnancy figure because you can appreciate all the benefits there are in having your body back every day. You can fit into your favorite pre-pregnancy clothes again, and even buy new ones in your usual size. You feel lighter and leaner, and probably more energetic as well. You'll want to continue to treat yourself well in relation to the food you eat and your entire lifestyle.

Small weight gains can happen to anyone, no matter how motivated you are. You might find a few pounds creeping back on during good times in your life—holidays, vacations—or during the stressful times that will always arise for parents. The best way to stay on top of the situation is to weigh yourself regularly—at least once a week—to monitor slight fluctuations and prevent them from becoming big gains. If you do gain more than a few pounds, you can just go right back on the Post-Pregnancy Diet for a week or two to lose them again. You know you can always lose weight on this diet because you've done it before; you already know how easy it is to stick to a diet that really works.

Getting back into the body you had before you became pregnant feels wonderful. More than any other change you might experience, regaining your pre-pregnancy figure can give you the very comfortable feeling that you're finally yourself again in the shape that you were before you became pregnant—the shape that you'll be keeping from now on!

Index

Meal plans (*Continued*)
  planning, 26
  weekends, 83–84
Meal scheduling, 25–26
  adapting, 122–23
  avoid eating child's leftovers, 116, 119
  child 1 to 3 months, 104–105
  child 3 to 6 months, 110–12
  child 6 to 12 months, 115–16
  child first to second year, 119
  child third year, 122–23
  family meal times, 112, 115, 119
  regular hours, 104–105
  rules for, 115, 119
  stay seated during meal, 115, 119
  supplemental snacks, 111
  working mothers, 110–11
Menus
  dinners, 52–68, 74–76
    Week 1, 52–60
    Week 2, 60–68
    five-day, 31–43
  lunches, 68–71
  restaurant meals, 26, 49, 71–76
Metabolism, 19–20, 21
Milk, 95, 96, 97
  reconstituted, 95
  skim, 96
"Mini-diet," 160
Mix-and-match selection charts, 72, 74–76
Mixed Brown Bag Lunch, 71
Motherhood, stages of, 101–24
  child from birth to 3 months, 102–108
    breast-feeding, 102–104
    fatigue, 105–107
    meal scheduling, 104–105
    your own time, 107–108
  child from third to sixth month, 108–13
    breast-feeding, 109–110
    fatigue, 112–13
    meal scheduling, 110–12
    your own time, 113
  child from 6 to 12 months, 114–18
    breast-feeding, 114–15
    fatigue, 116–17
    meal scheduling, 115–16
    your own time, 117–18
  child's first to second year, 118–21
    breast-feeding, 118–19
    fatigue, 119–20
    meal scheduling, 119
    your own time, 120–21

child's third year, 121–24
    breast-feeding, 122
    fatigue, 123–24
    meal scheduling, 122–23
    time on your own, 124
  exercises, 125–26
    first stage, 129–32
    second stage, 132–44
    third stage, 145–51
    video recommendations, 151–56
Motivation to diet, 49, 161
Mozzarella cheese
  part-skim, 51
  Salad Dijonnaise, 94
Mushrooms
  Mushroom Mug, 81
  Shrimp and Mushroom Toss, 67

Natural foods, 14, 96
New Mom's Milkshake, 9–10, 29, 77, 78, 79
  breast-feeding moms, 77, 78, 79, 103–104
  nutrients, 103
  recipe, 43
  working mothers, 111
Nursing mothers *see* Breast-feeding
Nutrition, 7, 10–12
  Post-Pregnancy Diet, 16, 19, 25, 26, 77–78

Osteoporosis, prevention of, 49
Overeating, 113

Paper-Wrapped Fish Fillets, 62–63
Parmesan Cauliflower, 55
Parmesan cheese, 15, 51
Pasta, 46, 90
  Cheese and Herb Pasta, 66–67
  Fettucine Primavera, 93
Pea Soup Snacks, 79
Peppers
  Stuffed Peppers Italiano, 56
Permitted Fruits list, 46–47, 73
Permitted Ingredients for Dinner Preparation, 44–45, 82, 97
Permitted Ingredients list, 17, 50
  wine included, 17
Physician's approval, 13, 22, 126, 129
  for exercise program, 22, 126, 129
Pita Jelly Fruit Roll, 80
Planning ahead, 74